The
In-Law
Survival Manu

The In-Law Survival Manual

A Guide
to
Cultivating
Healthy
In-Law Relationships

Gloria Call Horsley, RN, MFCC

JOHN WILEY & SONS, INC.

New York • Chichester • Brisbane • Toronto • Singapore • Weinheim

To Phil

Cover photograph: Chris Shorten
Illustrations: Gena Alder

This text is printed on acid-free paper.

Library of Congress Cataloging-in-Publication Data:

Horsley, Gloria Call.
    The in-law survival manual : a guide to cultivating healthy in-law relationships / by Gloria Call Horsley.
      p.   cm.
    Includes bibliographical references.
    ISBN 0-471-14963-2 (pbk. : alk. paper)
    1. Parents-in-law.   2. Parent and adult child.   3. Family.
I. Title.
HQ759.8.H67   1996
646.7'8—dc20   96-20521

Printed in the United States of America

10 9 8 7 6 5 4 3 2 1

Preface

In-law relationships present an interesting paradox. Although they have unlimited potential to cause problems, these relationships, when accorded the attention they deserve, also can add great joy to people's lives. Many of us feel uncomfortable in any interaction with our in-laws; we may even have an *us-versus-them* mentality. The in-law relationship represents an unaddressed problem area, yet it has far-reaching implications for individuals and couples.

Because in-law problems are so deeply embedded in the fiber of the family unit, they are often not recognized for what they are. People seem to view in-law problems as they do weeds: they are less than attractive, but they are not likely to kill anyone. However, embedded within these harmless-looking relationships can be the seeds of destruction and malignancy. In time, if allowed to gestate, they can produce new and extended growth of long-standing root systems. Any gardener who has diligently torn out old plantings will still find a surviving weed, or even a beautiful flower, popping up in the same spot during the next season.

People seem to view in-law problems as they do weeds.

During more than a decade of individual and family counseling, I have observed that, without proactive steps to strengthen and continue to build on positive in-law communications, clients may unwittingly propagate undesirable relationships with the extended family. When new or historical contacts with in-laws are fraught with pain and distress, extended family members eventually find themselves less able to be together cordially, which fosters a deliberate distancing from the family—or what Dr. Murray Bowen called *emotional cutoffs*.

My experience during more than 15 years of therapy with individuals, couples, and their extended families has taught me that the in-law connection does not have to be that way. With time and maturity, we can

Learn to use the extended family as a resource.

learn to use the extended family as a resource—and a base for mutually fulfilling relationships.

Toward Healthy In-Law Relationships

The purpose of my work is not to define how people should act and behave; rather, I give suggestions for ideas that might effect change within ourselves, thus bringing about change in our extended family. I have written this book to create an opportunity for talking about in-law issues by observing how others creatively work out their in-law problems.

One individual cannot be expected to change an entire family.

One individual cannot be expected to change an entire family. This book is about how *you can change yourself* within the in-law system, how you can adjust your own attitudes and behaviors toward your extended family. Throughout the book, you will be offered opportunities to ask yourself, "What can I do to change myself? What can I do to change my expectations of my in-laws and other family members, given that they may choose not to change?"

In-Law Relationships: Where Are We?

This book calls for a major shift in dealing with in-laws, and identifies ways to improve your in-law relationships. Building good in-law relationships can help you add a depth and breadth to your life that you may not otherwise have. The analogy of hearty broth has often been used to represent families. In a parallel analogy, I would suggest that the *in-law family* is a *family stew*. The ingredients are blended together, but each maintains its own flavor and individuality.

Find some useful tools for starting new in-law relationships.

I hope this book will help you to find some useful tools for starting new in-law relationships on the right foot and then keeping them strong. If your in-law relationships are already out of kilter, the book provides practical techniques to help you move them back into balance. The book's advice may create a dialogue between and among family members, which may allow your family to redefine its in-law problems. And, for families already enjoying good in-law relationships, this book may show that you deserve a pat on the back because you have avoided the many pitfalls of being an in-law.

GLORIA CALL HORSLEY

San Francisco, California

Acknowledgments

I would like to acknowledge Phil, my husband of 36 years, for his enthusiastic support of my writing.

I thank Heidi and Mark Redding, Rebecca and John Bara, and Heather and Shawn Johnson, my three daughters and their husbands, for their encouragement and ideas. And, God bless my grandchildren, Eliza and Scott Bara, and the soon-to-arrive Johnson baby. Their hugs and kisses keep their grandma going. I also acknowledge the silent support of our son, Scott, who, although no longer with us, continues to be a strong force in our lives.

Thanks to Peter Wiley for his encouragement and publishing insight.

Deep appreciation is extended to Beverly McManus, my friend and editor, for her excellent editorial skills and her constant reminder that writing a book is really fun. Thanks also to her husband, Steve, and her daughters, Emily and Mary Ella, for sharing Beverly's creative energy.

Thanks to Karen Lau, who stuck with us for a second book. Her fleet fingers, speed, and accuracy, along with her unfailing good humor, are much appreciated. Thanks also to her daughters, Erin and Denise, for their loving support of their mother.

Thanks to Kelly Franklin, my fabulous editor at Wiley, whose ideas, creativity, and strategic support have made working together on this second in-law book so rewarding. Kudos to Nancy Marcus Land for her enthusiastic and detailed copy editing.

Thanks to Gena Alder for her creative graphic support.

Thanks to Steve Alder and the Health Research Center at the University of Utah, for statistical analysis of my in-law research data.

Appreciation goes to Chris Shorten for his photographic talents.

And thanks to Dr. Florence Kaslow, who encouraged me to put my thoughts and the content of my practice into a book.

I also am deeply indebted to the pioneering research of Dr. Evelyn Duvall, who, more than 40 years ago, launched one of the only explorations into the in-law relationship.

Thanks go to Dr. Marguerite McCorkle, Director of Research at the Mental Research Institute (MRI), Palo Alto, California, for her assistance in designing my in-law research.

Thanks to my supportive friends and colleagues. A special thanks to Trev Blazzard for his insight into in-law legal, financial, and due diligence issues. And thanks to Fanita English for her insight into in-law communication.

I am especially thankful for my grandmother, Mamie Peters Call, who raised her ten children and still found time to write five books. Thanks also to Joan and Richard Haskins, Bill and Mary Call, Reed and Marilyn Walker, and Margaret Watson, who, as siblings and siblings-in-law, fill my heart with joy and delight.

And last but not least, thanks to my friends, family, and clients, whose in-law stories fill this book.

G.C.H.

Contents

PART FOUR

MENDING FENCES

PART ONE

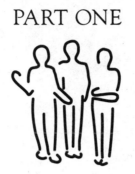

TYPES OF IN-LAWS

1

What Type of In-Law Are You?

A New View of the In-Law Continuum: From Toxic Agents to A Pain in the Neck to Tolerance, and Even Love

Being an in-law is different from being a friend or neighbor. Maintaining cordial or even civil in-law connections over a lifetime can be difficult. Sometimes, family members or new in-laws have lost the battle before they even knew they were in a fight.

In-law problems and relationships cannot all be painted with the same brush—the solutions to them are unique and filled with as much variety as the people they represent. However, in the pages that follow are some ideas—a synthesis of my observations of many hundreds of families plus the input of a number of preeminent family therapists—on how you might think about yourself in terms of your in-laws.

Unique solutions are needed

This book will help you understand the stages of in-law relationships by looking at some in-law relationships that work and some that do not. It will help you explore the secrets of in-law relationships and offer some ideas on what you can expect from your in-laws.

Being a successful in-law is worth the effort. Whether a parent-in-law, child-in-law, sibling-in-law, or ex-in-law, each person within a family system has the opportunity to add richness—or sorrow—to the relationship.

Assess your in-law relationship with each individual in-law.

I have a particular interest in telling you how to deal with your *in-law* rather than your in-laws, because people seldom have problems with their in-laws en masse; instead, a specific in-law or small group of in-laws is the source of conflict. Remedies become particularly difficult when you think about your in-laws. "Her parents do this," or "His parents do that." "My in-laws do this, my in-laws do that." Are all your in-laws really doing whatever offends you, or is just one in-law persisting in a behavior that you do not like? To improve in-law relationships, you have to focus your activities on improving bonds with one in-law at a time. This book can help you clarify and assess your in-law relationship with each individual in-law.

Long-term, deep-seated family problems are difficult for families to face; as an in-law, you may have to skirt around them. Building strong in-law relationships requires a great deal of energy, as well as desire. With some of the exercises and concepts in this book, you will be better able to deal with intrafamily problems or even to avoid them altogether. When in-law relationships are kept clear of hostilities and resentments, mutually satisfying interactions are possible—with even the most difficult relatives. As we age and family members pass away, our resources diminish. It therefore seems prudent to maximize all available resources, especially those within the family circle. By changing *your* attitudes, you can go a long way toward helping family members to value their in-law relationships and to deal with in-laws wisely and kindly.

In-Laws—An Odd Space between Friends and Relatives

In-laws represent an undefined web of relationships.

Your in-laws are an intricate and basic part of your spouse's or partner's history, although they in many ways represent an unacknowledged, undefined web of relationships. One day, on the way to the airport, a cab driver opined that people don't relate as much to in-law relationships because biological relationships are more primal. He added, "In my family, I have seen my spouse automatically rally to her brother's defense if I criticize him. In a way, this gives me comfort, because I know she would do the same for me." As this cab driver saw it, "In-laws fall in this odd space between friends and relatives."

As an in-law or potential in-law, you have the power to decide how you will fill that space between friends and relatives. Will the space be filled with friendly words, kind deeds, loving acts, and caring behaviors? Will it be filled with pride for accomplishments, support for failure as well as success, understanding of faults and slights because you are able to see in-laws in a different light? Or will the in-law space be filled with contention, animosity, disappointment, and jealousy?

In-laws fall in this odd space between friends and relatives.

Building Successful In-Law Relationships

In the United States today, approximately 2.4 million couples marry each year. If we take into consideration the fact that a majority of the *parents* of these newlyweds are still living, this means there are upward of 9,600,000 new in-law relationships created every year—and this accounts for only the parents of the children who married, who, throughout this book, are referred to as *parents-in-law*. I refer to those 2.4 million who marry as *children-in-law*, because, with their marriages, each becomes a son- or daughter-in-law to the spouse's parents. Just imagine how large the number would grow if we were to consider brothers- and sisters-in-law (referred to throughout this book as *siblings-in-law*), as well as stepfamilies and *quasi-in-laws* (parents and relatives of couples who are living together but are not married). In *The Wife-in-Law Trap*, Ann Cryster has extended the in-law web to include her ex-husband's second wife, whom she terms the *wife-in-law*. Where divorces and remarriages have occurred, the number of potential in-laws soars exponentially.

Upward of 9,600,000 new in-law relationships created every year.

Monica McGoldrick, a social worker with the Family Institute of Westchester and a well-known family therapist and author, sees the majority of marital problems as carryovers from unresolved extended family

The majority of marital problems are carryovers from extended family problems.

problems. In her experiences with families, unresolved family issues are often significant factors in marital choice. With the divorce rate in the United States approaching 50 percent of all marriages, it would seem that if you and your in-laws want the marriage to work, you are best advised to try to work out issues as early as possible in the relationship.

According to Evelyn R. Duvall, who in 1954 researched in-law relationships and wrote a book on her findings, becoming a good in-law is a lifelong task for all of us.

If you want to get along better with your in-laws, your best approach is to start with yourself.

If you want to get along better with your in-laws, your best approach is to start with yourself. The first question you should ask yourself is what kind of in-law are you or do you want to be?

How Do You View the World?

Each of us has a unique view of the world, and this view tends to influence how we react to the circumstances we encounter. Many models of personality types have been developed to help us determine who we are and understand how we see things. One of the most useful models is the Enneagram, which divides people into nine different personality types. I have adapted the Enneagram types to the following in-law types to help you and your in-laws explore how each of you looks at the world:

1. The Critical In-Law.

2. The Giving In-Law.

3. The Superachieving In-Law.

4. The Emotionally Intense In-Law.

5. The Observant In-Law.

6. The Opposing-View In-Law.

7. The Gadabout In-Law.

8. The Take-Charge In-Law.

9. The Conflict-Avoidance In-Law.

The types of behaviors that you are drawn to impact your relationships with your in-laws. We all have a wish to be loved, noticed, and accepted. In-laws sometimes have strange and unique ways of acknowledging our wish or demanding that their own wish be given priority.

The questionnaire on pages 8–12 will help you to distinguish your own characteristics and to give you better insight into what motivates your in-law behaviors.

Some clients find it hard to determine their in-law type. Descriptions of each of the in-law types might seem to apply equally to any given individual, but the descriptions for *only one* of the in-law types will typically strike a very deep chord for each person. There is a *good news/bad news* precept for in-laws (as well as for most human relationships). The bad news is that you cannot change your in-laws. The good news is that you can change yourself. If you change yourself, the relationship with your in-laws has to change, too. Hence, when you are experiencing conflicts with your in-laws, it is helpful to first identify your own personality type, then determine how each of your in-laws views the world.

Complete these questions and, if possible, compare your answers with your in-laws'. You may find that you and an in-law share a similar world-view; or, you may be surprised at how different you really are.

The Critical In-Law

Critical, or even hypercritical, in-laws are people who know how all of the adults and children in the family (as well as the universe) should behave. Miss Manners and Emily Post are their gurus. They love to be right, *The critical in-law loves to be right.*

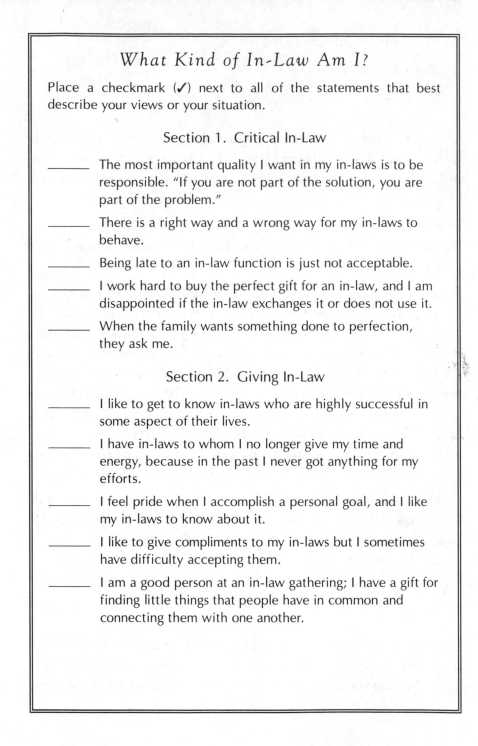

What Kind of In-Law Am I?

Place a checkmark (✓) next to all of the statements that best describe your views or your situation.

Section 1. Critical In-Law

_____ The most important quality I want in my in-laws is to be responsible. "If you are not part of the solution, you are part of the problem."

_____ There is a right way and a wrong way for my in-laws to behave.

_____ Being late to an in-law function is just not acceptable.

_____ I work hard to buy the perfect gift for an in-law, and I am disappointed if the in-law exchanges it or does not use it.

_____ When the family wants something done to perfection, they ask me.

Section 2. Giving In-Law

_____ I like to get to know in-laws who are highly successful in some aspect of their lives.

_____ I have in-laws to whom I no longer give my time and energy, because in the past I never got anything for my efforts.

_____ I feel pride when I accomplish a personal goal, and I like my in-laws to know about it.

_____ I like to give compliments to my in-laws but I sometimes have difficulty accepting them.

_____ I am a good person at an in-law gathering; I have a gift for finding little things that people have in common and connecting them with one another.

What Kind of In-Law Am I?
(Continued)

Section 3. Superachieving In-Law

_____ I like my in-laws to think well of me, and I will go out of my way to do something helpful, even though I really do not have time.

_____ I sometimes have to cut corners or be late when helping in-laws, because I tend to overcommit.

_____ My in-laws are amazed at my ability to complete a number of tasks.

_____ I can sometimes be rude to or ignore an individual family member in order to complete an assignment.

_____ I almost always have goals when I visit my in-laws. In that way, I have not wasted my day.

Section 4. Emotionally Intense In-Law

_____ Being seen as a unique and special in-law is important to me.

_____ I see myself as a person with an artistic and sensitive nature.

_____ I tend to choose clothes or have items in my home that have special meaning to me.

_____ I am a great listener to in-laws who have problems, especially if they have experienced a loss.

_____ Sometimes, I feel a sense of envy at the talents or material things that my in-laws have.

Section 5. Observant In-Law

_____ My in-laws sometimes see me as standoffish, and it is true that intrusive people bother me.

(continued)

What Kind of In-Law Am I?
(Continued)

_____ I enjoy thinking about pleasant in-law experiences more after they happen than during the event.

_____ I watch in-law interactions and often choose not to get involved; however, if in-laws approach me for help with problem in-laws, I have many good ideas.

_____ I really feel that I am a bit smarter than the majority of my in-laws.

_____ I do not mind not being asked to bring anything to in-law functions. I think my being there is enough.

Section 6. Opposing-View In-Law

_____ When talking to my in-laws, I tend to take the role of devil's advocate, seeing the other side of most issues.

_____ I remember when an in-law has slighted me or put me down, and then I do everything in my power to avoid him or her.

_____ I measure myself against other in-laws and can become self-doubting and fearful.

_____ I do not really trust in-laws whom I do not know well; it is a dangerous world.

_____ I get nervous around in-laws whom I view as authority figures.

Section 7. The Gadabout In-Law

_____ I hate to be tied down (committed) to spending every Sunday or holiday with my in-laws. So many things are possible; I like to keep my options open.

_____ I tend to avoid in-laws who dwell too much on the negative. I tell them to turn lemons into lemonade.

What Kind of In-Law Am I?
(Continued)

_____ Depressed in-laws are people whom I do not have time for. Depression is contagious. If an in-law is depressed, I tell him or her to just get over it.

_____ I do not enjoy sitting and talking with my in-laws. My idea of fun is when we have a lot of activities or projects planned.

_____ I like it when my in-laws do things in a classy way. Second-rate events or accommodations are not my style.

Section 8. The Take-Charge In-Law

_____ Some in-laws see me as pushy, but when an activity involves me, I am good at telling people what to do.

_____ I respect in-laws who tell me face-to-face if they have a problem with me.

_____ I am known as the in-law who will not take any nonsense.

_____ In-laws can depend on me to stand up for them if they need help.

_____ I can get angry, and on more than one occasion my anger has gotten out of hand

Section 9. The Conflict-Avoidance In-Law

_____ If things get too boring or tense with my in-laws, I will leave the situation mentally, read a magazine, or go for a walk.

_____ I like to talk to one in-law at a time. In that way, I can really get into what each one is doing with his or her life.

_____ I am able to see both sides of the issue when my in-laws have disputes. This is why my in-laws often turn to me to help them resolve tiffs.

(continued)

> ## What Kind of In-Law Am I?
> ### (Continued)
>
> _____ My in-laws may see me as low-key, but I am actually an intense person. Still waters run deep.
>
> _____ I see myself as being an open-minded in-law.
>
> *Scoring:* Add up the number of statements you checked in each section. The sections with the most checks may give you clues to your in-law personality type. If you have equal numbers of checks in two or more sections, read on. The overview of each in-law type should help you to clarify who you are and how you see the world.

and often are. They hold themselves (as well as their in-laws and their siblings) to a high standard. Most of them hate being late, and they expect family gatherings to be at the right place and the right time. They can become quite angry, especially if they feel that they are right and others are not meeting their standards. Critical in-laws can be very direct in their anger; they speak from the gut, and often will not remember what they have said to offend their in-laws. The best ways of getting along with critical in-laws are: try to be on time, and do what you have promised to do. If you are upset with a critical in-law, confront him or her directly—but in private.

The Giving In-Law

The giving in-law speaks from the heart.

Giving in-laws often speak from the heart. Early in the in-law relationship, they will listen to what the new in-law says and will give a great deal of attention and largesse to both the new in-law and his or her spouse. However, if they give a lot and do not feel that they have been given enough in return, they may cut off the offending party and become somewhat cold. This turnabout may be aggravating to the person who has been cut off, because the giving in-laws will have close and cozy relationships with other in-laws or family members. Giving in-laws gravitate toward powerful people and enjoy sharing someone else's spotlight. These in-laws can be prideful and require a great deal of attention. Despite looking provocative, flirtatious, and dependent at times, they are very independent people. Giving in-laws tend to be very high-energy people. They are creative and playful, and they know how to have a good time. If you have giving in-laws, make sure to acknowledge their kindnesses—and return the favor by taking an interest in them. Do not be put off by bursts of temper from giving in-laws. They are basically loving people who are willing to forgive and forget. Spend time having fun and laughing with them, but also take an interest in their problems.

The Superachieving In-Law

This is the American prototype of the successful in-law—someone who is always working on projects, whether at the office or at home. This in-law takes a to-do list on vacation. At home, major projects may include building fences or hooking room-size rugs. This in-law is always trying to show how successful he or she is, to impress the parents-in-law. After Thanksgiving dinner, this super sibling is in the kitchen washing dishes or has just finished carving the leftover turkey and is starting to make sandwiches. The superachiever irritates other take-charge siblings-in-law by bossing them around. This constant drive for competition and pats on the back can drive the other siblings and in-laws crazy, because their parents always compare them with the super sibling. A super sibling is a Type-A personality who often ends up with health problems or in family crisis as a result of never having any downtime.

The super-achieving in-law is always working on projects.

If you have superachieving in-laws, let them know that you like them for who they are and not just for what they achieve. Point out when they are working too hard and not taking care of their health.

The Emotionally Intense In-Law

The emotionally intense in-law experiences a depth of feelings.

Emotionally intense-in-laws often have comfortable and unique home environments. They may have distinctive ways of dressing and enjoy being a little off beat, with eclectic clothing or an unusual haircut. They are intense people and like to think and talk about the tragedies of the world. They feel special because they can experience a depth of feelings that others do not have. They understand and know loss. They are aware that the world is not complete, and they long for what is missing. These in-laws can be jealous of siblings as well as other in-laws, but will often express this jealousy in passive-aggressive ways, such as being late for events or complaining about the work created by the family reunion, which they planned. They rarely delegate; instead, they constantly *do*, in order to be praised as the special people they are. Emotionally intense in-laws may be problematic for brothers-in-law and sisters-in-law because they want to have deep emotional relationships; however, there is ambivalence because they also envy the close relationship the in-law (husband, wife) has with their sibling. These in-laws constantly get in trouble by telling people their *real* feelings. They can be difficult to live with. They get too deeply into their emotions, going at times too high, too low, too deep, or too far out. When they go too deep, severe depression can result.

If you have an emotionally intense in-law, appreciate the fact that he or she feels strongly about the beauty and drama of life. Accept the propensity toward depression; however, if you think the in-law is going too deep into the dark side of life, point it out and encourage him or her to lighten up.

The Observant In-Law

The observant in-law lives in a world of ideas.

These in-laws tend to be real loners and thinkers. They enjoy sitting back and observing the family, rather than being actively engaged in its activities. Although they are often seen as shy and withdrawn, they really like living in their world of ideas. To explore these ideas, they require time to think about and process family events. For example, they will enjoy their sister-in-law's concert far more after the event, when they have gone home and have had time to contemplate and replay the event in their heads. These in-laws carefully guard their time and energy—and often their money—because they fear that these resources are in short supply. Because of their tendency to withdraw, they can become isolated and are often overlooked by the more active in-laws. They expect that other family members also enjoy being left alone; however, this respect for others' privacy can be mistaken for a lack of interest in family issues. They are often highly dependent on the family network because they do not interact with many people. They may work in jobs that are isolated, such as computer analysis or accounting. When approached, they tend to be sensitive and caring and can be good people to go to with problems. Many are logical, knowledgeable, and original thinkers.

If you have an observant in-law, respect his or her choice to watch rather than be involved in family games. Be sensitive to the fact that even though this person might not be the life of the party, family and in-laws are an important part of his or her life. Do not be afraid to give an occasional hug—this in-law needs to be encouraged to express emotion.

The Opposing-View In-Law

Some in-laws are crazy-making: they always take the opposite view on every statement that an in-law makes. These in-laws are often caught up in causes and are a bit paranoid about those who do not agree with their opinions. Because they are self-doubting and take the devil's advocate role, they may have trouble staying with a tough situation or making a decision. They seem to be lying in wait for an in-law to make a mistake or to slight them. When it happens, they have a feeling of satisfaction because it is the proof that they have been looking for, the evidence that their in-law does not like or respect them after all. They are constantly

The opposing-view in-law constantly scans the in-law environment.

scanning the in-law environment for dangerous, sabotaging in-laws. They are hypersensitive to slights. "Yes, my brother-in-law didn't ask me to usher at his wedding." They relish holding a grudge. These in-laws can be powerhouses in the family. Often, they are the people who can be relied on to carry out difficult and time-consuming projects. If you have a good cause, you can count on them to take up the banner. If you're saving the spotted owl or the whales, they are with you.

If you have an opposing-view in-law and enjoy a heated discussion, argue with the opposing-view in-law. He or she will love it and is good at it. However, do not make fun of a passion for causes; they are very important to this in-law. Also, make sure you do not overpromise; you will be expected to come through and to deliver more than good intentions.

The Gadabout In-Law

The gadabout in-law is in constant search for all of the experiences life offers.

These in-laws have been called human hummingbirds. They are always on the go—constantly searching for all of the experiences that life has to offer. Their running around is based in a fear that they will be stuck in depression or despair if they stop. Thus, their modus operandi is constant activity. They invite you to stay for a week but do not cancel any of their usual activities. They invite you along or they leave you at home with their kids "so they can get to know Auntie." Gadabouts can be fun to have for in-laws, but they can also be frustrating. They are always looking for the best option and, late on Saturday night, they may decide that Sunday dinner with you is not high on their agenda. They always have a lot of tasks going and may only need to complete a few. This can be frustrating: it may be *your* job they do not get done. They are masters at getting others to do their work.

If you have a gadabout in-law, try not to get frustrated with the inevitable flurry of ideas and activity. Be aware that staying in perpetual motion helps him or her not to become fearful. If you are clear about the dates and times that you need him or her available, the gadabout will usually comply. This is a loyal family member.

The Take-Charge In-Law

This is the in-law who always needs to be in charge of every situation, is easily pissed-off, and at times seems like a bully. This in-law does not mind a good argument and is often surprised when an in-law has been offended by the energy of a response. Alcohol and the take-charge in-law often do not mix. This person can not only take charge, but may completely run over everybody else, causing in-law rifts that are difficult to mend. Although at times this person seems overbearing, his or her assertiveness is excellent for moving people and groups forward. This in-law will pull together huge family reunions and, through sheer energy, will make sure everyone has fun (possibly with a few arguments along the way). This is a courageous leader who inspires others to speak their own mind.

The take-charge in-law always needs to move people a certain way.

If you have a take-charge in-law, you need to point out when the argument or discussion is getting too heated for you by making *I'm feeling uncomfortable* statements. When things get too uncomfortable, excuse yourself. There is no point in trying to talk down an angry take-charge in-law.

The Conflict-Avoidance In-Law

These in-laws can see all sides of an argument. They are great to talk to, and they give good advice regarding problems with other in-laws or with spouses. They can be trusted to keep a secret. These in-laws appear to be very good-natured and seem to have all the time in the world for other people's problems, all the while ignoring their own problems that are churning inside. Conflict-avoidance in-laws will put the petty problems

The conflict-avoidance in-law lets inessentials crowd out essentials.

of others above their own, which often may not be so petty, such as finding a job or following through on their child's request. They can lose focus and let inessentials crowd out essentials. Conflict-avoidance in-laws may space out on food, TV, books, or alcohol. Conflict avoiders are wonderful in-laws, but if they let their anger go to sleep and avoid dealing with problems, their anger and resentment may explosively erupt when least expected. Remember, they are much deeper and more intelligent than one may think. Underneath that easy-going facade is a highly competitive and very stubborn in-law.

If you have a conflict-avoidance in-law, remember that his or her opinions on family events and activities can easily be overlooked. If you want this person to be involved, it is important to pass along information, ask for opinions, and then follow through on the suggestions given. You'll be treated fairly and reasonably if you express respect and understanding. Acknowledge this in-law's needs and allow *down time* for recharging his or her batteries.

How Knowledge of the In-Law Points-of-View Can Help You to Work Out Relationship Conflicts

The nine in-law types are very different—not inherently *bad* or *good*, just different. When you figure out what type of in-law you are—and realize that your in-laws may have a different point of view—the understanding you gain regarding differences will help you build a good relationship and overcome the problems and obstacles all in-laws face.

If you are still not sure what type you are, take the time to fill out the worksheet at the end of this chapter. There are some defining questions about your childhood that will help you determine your in-law type.

It may seem clear to you that, in the long run, it is in everyone's best interest to work out in-law relationships. But you may wonder: "How is this done? How do I work on getting along with my in-law? Do I ignore all the conflicts, and hope that maturity will prevail? Do I take the subject up with his or her spouse or parents-in-law and risk creating a conflict in the clan? Or do I confront the in-law directly?" These are difficult questions, and I hope you will find more answers as you read the subsequent chapters.

Now that you have a general idea of your in-law personality type, keep it in mind as you read the rest of the book. One of the most important aspects of knowing your type is being aware that other in-laws have a different way of viewing the world. They are not just trying to get your goat. They really do not see things through your lens.

Worksheet

If you still have not figured out what type of in-law you are, review the following questions, which are based on your childhood. The one that strikes the most chords should give you an indication of your in-law type.

1. **The critical in-law.** Were your early behaviors primarily targeted to avoid criticism and punishment through correct behavior? Are you convinced there is only one right way to do any task?

2. **The giving in-law.** Was your acceptance in the family based on your ability to please others? As a child did you draw attention to yourself by being cute or charming?

3. **The superachieving in-law.** Was your value in the family predicated on your performance? Do you think that in order to be recognized and liked you must complete projects?

4. **The emotionally intense in-law.** Did you feel abandoned or suffer a real or imagined loss in your early years from which you have never fully recovered? Does *melancholy* describe your inner emotions? Do you have a sense that things could and should be better than they are here and now?

(continued)

Worksheet
(Continued)

5. **The observant in-law.** Was it necessary to develop a rich inner world to protect your personal self and feelings from attack and to have your individual opinions and values respected? Are time and energy your most important assets, which you must guard from others?

6. **The opposing-view in-law.** As a child, was your home life and the discipline you received unpredictable? To avoid being hurt or embarrassed, was it important to check out danger signals in your home and then change your behavior accordingly?

7. **The gadabout in-law.** Do you have a positive memory of your childhood, even though you objectively had somewhat less than happy experiences? Do you move toward pleasure and away from pain?

8. **The take-charge in-law.** Did you feel dominated by bigger, stronger people who wanted to control your life? As a child, did your survival depend on being strong and taking a tough, personal stand in any confrontation?

9. **The conflict-avoidance in-law.** Did you have to hide your anger and opinions in order to be heard or accepted by your parents? Were your feelings and priorities discounted, causing you to abandon your own point of view and take on the opinions of others?

2

Bad In-Laws and Good In-Laws

One of the keys to having good in-law relationships is to have realistic expectations. All families have different expectations of how the in-law relationship will work. This chapter looks into the different *roles* you may fill as an in-law: the parent-in-law, the child-in-law, and the sibling-in-law. If all the jokes, stories, and myths about in-laws are to be believed, there are countless ways to be a bad in-law. Simply by not trying, *anyone* can be a bad in-law. In the short term, it may seem attractive to be a horrible in-law—to let it rip, regardless of the consequences. In the long run, however, relationships are more satisfying when participants thoughtfully consider the consequences of their actions and are willing to be flexible and to withhold criticism. As you review the bad in-law actions described here, you will note a pattern of selfish, hostile, and needy behaviors.

There are countless ways to be a bad in-law.

Following this overview of ways to be an ugly in-law, we will look at some of the qualities that can be fostered for the development of healthy in-law relationships.

Five Actions That Can Make You a Bad Parent-In-Law

1. *Take every opportunity to give advice and criticism.*

You can make lots of mistakes as a parent-in-law by not asking what other people want, and assuming that you already know. These assumptions are often based on what you think your in-laws should be doing, rather than on what they want to do.

Each of us has our own pace and style of working that needs to be respected. We also have our own ideas about how a family should be run. If you force your opinion on your in-laws, you have to deal with the consequences when they discover it was the wrong solution.

2. *Make sure that you pin the children-in-law down as to the specific reasons they are missing a family event.*

Explore opportunities to meet your needs outside of the family.

You have your right to live and plan your own life. Do your in-laws have that same right? You can make your in-laws feel very guilty when they pursue their own needs. As a parent-in-law, you can be very needy and often angry because your needs are not being met. If you do not want to be this way, explore opportunities to meet your needs outside of the family and to connect with your children in a less needy way. When children-in-law decline your invitation, they can get into trouble by giving too much *free information*, as in the following telephone conversation:

PARENT-IN-LAW: "Will you join us for dinner on Sunday?"

CHILD-IN-LAW: "Sorry, can't make it. We are going to get together with some friends from work and then I have to wash my car and network on the computer." (Too much information.)

PARENT-IN-LAW: "Well, why don't you give me a call when you can fit us into your busy schedule." (Hangs up.)

This conversation can work both ways; when in-laws are given too much information, it is natural for them to make a judgment on the behavior. If your in-laws are hassling you about priorities, you might respond with, "Sorry, we can't make it. We have previous commitments."

3. *Tell in-laws that you will help them out financially, and then don't do it.*

When possible, say "Yes."

As a parent-in-law, you have a right to be ambiguous in your communications, even if you risk offending your children-in-law. Bear in mind, however, that this ambiguity can be very confusing to newcomers to the family. I advise parents-in-law who cannot help out, or choose not to, to say "No." Say it clearly, say it politely; but say it. Do not lead your in-laws into believing that you are going to act for them when you are not. They would much rather know that you are not going to contribute than have a false impression that you are going to help them out. Also, when possible, say "Yes." You need opportunities to say yes to your in-laws and to help them as best you can. In-laws may avoid coming to you if you always say no and then have to be talked into doing something. If you think you might want to do it, say yes right away.

4. *Criticize the disciplining of grandchildren.*

The topic of discipline of children is rife with opportunities to be a bad in-law. Grandparents seldom have the same expectations that parents do about children's behavior. Disagreements most often arise because the grandparents have disregarded the boundaries of the parents/children unit. Either they intrude into an area where they do not belong, or they encourage the grandchildren to disobey the parents, with the excuse that "It's fun to spoil our grandchildren—we see them so seldom, what can it hurt?" This emotionally laden area deserves its own chapter (see Chapter 5).

The grandparents have disregarded the boundaries of the parents.

5. *Try to control everyone and everything, including putting signs above the faucets with arrows telling the users which way to turn them on and off.*

Why increase your flexibility with regard to differences in opinions and attitudes? It is much more fun to be a rigid, controlling parent-in-law. Understanding anothers' side of an issue does not mean that you must agree with them. You can have your own opinions and let your in-laws have theirs. Before you take a harsh stand with a new in-law, take a moment to consider your options—and the possible consequences—if the outcome is not to your liking. Sometimes, helping behaviors are actually ways to control others. As a parent-in-law, wait to be asked before you insist on jumping in to help your child-in-law.

You can have your own opinions and let your in-laws have theirs.

Five Ways to Be a Horrible Child-in-Law

Following are five actions that, I assure you, will make you a horrible child-in-law. You can add to the list and identify some unique causes of friction in your family.

1. *Refuse to visit.*

A way of punishing your spouse by not spending time with his or her family.

One tactic that is guaranteed to annoy everyone is a refusal to visit your in-laws. This may be a snub or a way of punishing your spouse by not spending time with his or her family. If you are punishing your in-laws by refusing to visit them, then this also punishes your children, who miss out on seeing their grandparents. If you are forced to visit the in-laws, sulk; make sure everyone knows how miserable you are. It will make everyone feel bad to have you around the house. Who cares if nobody is quite sure what you are angry about? Keep 'em guessing!

2. *Borrow money and then do not pay it back.*

Families have broken apart or experienced turmoil because of unresolved money issues.

Borrowing money is a touchy subject with anyone, but especially with in-laws. It is easy when you are out and about together to say offhandedly, "Hey, have you got $20?" Some nice in-law pulls the $20 out of a purse or wallet and says, "Sure, here," and then you conveniently forget to pay it back. If you let it go a long time, this in-law probably will forget that you ever borrowed the money. Financial disputes are all too common among in-laws, and countless families have broken apart or experienced turmoil because of unresolved money issues. (More on this volatile topic in Chapter 11.)

3. *Leave your children with the in-laws, then do not return when you said you would.*

Why not take in a bargain matinee as long as the kids were left at Grandma's for the morning? She always says she cannot get enough of them! You can get away with this at least three or four times before Grandma catches on and puts her foot down.

Parents-in-law have varying attitudes about taking care of grandchildren. However, most of them have in common a desire to be asked whether they would *like* to take care of the children, and then they want to know what time you will be leaving, what time you will be back, and what the children's schedules are.

4. *Do not take their advice, or do take it, and then hold the in-laws forever responsible if it does not work out.*

As a child-in-law, you can feel very comfortable being like the majority of people, who generally do not follow other people's advice. If you make a decision that goes in the direction of an in-law's advice and it does not work out, you can put an in-law in a great deal of hot water and make him or her feel very guilty. If you are cunning, your in-laws may even be held responsible for your own decisions.

5. *Avoid sending thank-you notes to in-laws or acknowledging their assistance.*

Your life is busy and your in-laws may not realize that, as far as you are concerned, *saying* "thank you" is enough. Your quiet exclamations may have gone unheard by those busily engaged in keeping events on target. But, do not feel too bad. Most children do not thank their parents for everything that goes on, particularly while they are living in the home and are dependent, so parents-in-law should not expect a switch when children marry, move out of the home, and come back to visit.

Your quiet exclamations may have gone unheard.

Once the shift is made, parents often believe they must now be thanked for things that were taken for granted in the past. Appreciation extended to in-laws goes a long way toward developing good relationships and having people feel good about doing more things for you, so if you are trying to be a bad child-in-law, relinquish any thoughts of sending thank-you notes or bringing flowers when you come to dinner. If you do acknowledge help you receive from an in-law, it will blow them away.

Five Things You Can Do to Be a Terrible Sibling-in-Law

1. *Borrow the car, then return it with an empty gas tank or a dent in the fender.*

Just like differing housecleaning standards, people have different standards about their cars.

Why rent or buy your own car when you can use your brother- or sister-in-laws' car at no cost? Should you borrow your in-laws' car, especially a very nice car that they take a lot of pride in? You might risk the chance that your in-laws will be aggravated at you if you eat in their car or transport your animals in their minivan. Just like differing housecleaning standards, people have different standards about their cars.

Insurance can also become an issue. Is the car insured for the person who is driving it? What happens if you end up denting one of the fenders or returning it with a gash in the upholstery? How will they deal with this? Is it worth the hassle? Will they ignore the insurance risk or will they simply say, "No, I don't loan out my car"? You can be a very annoying sibling-in-law if you are unwilling to face up to your responsibilities.

2. *Cut down your sibling-in-laws whenever possible.*

In our society, badmouthing one's in-laws and talking negatively about them seems to be a rather enjoyable pastime. Some people cannot talk enough about how much they dislike their mother-in-law or brother-in-law or father-in-law or sister-in-law and what a pain in the neck the in-laws are and how they wish they did not have to deal with them. Often, people will rehash the same in-law grievances over and over again. This is sure to cause a lot of friction and deep rifts in the in-law relationship.

3. *Watch TV when they come to visit.*

One sure way to show your in-laws that you do not care about them is to watch TV when they come to visit. Because of their divergent interests, your in-laws may not be interested in watching the programs you enjoy. When they visit you, they expect they will get some attention, or at least some polite conversation. But why miss your favorite line-up on Thursday night just because your in-laws show up?

4. *Try to seduce your brother's wife.*

When siblings-in-law have affairs with each other, intense problems are created because after the affair breaks off, the in-law relationship remains. One cannot be a dance-away lover when one has to sit next to the ex-paramour at Thanksgiving dinner. Such was the dilemma expressed by my client, Natasha,* who had an affair with her brother-in-law, Bradley, a doctor, while her daughter was hospitalized for leukemia. She said, "It was only natural that I would look to a family member for support. Bradley was always there at the hospital, and we were thrown together in our grief and fear. All of a sudden, we started thinking we were in love and, since life was so short, we should do something about it. We ended the affair soon after Brittany was released from the hospital. The problem is, I can't stand to see Bradley at family events now because it reminds me of how I have betrayed my family."

What if you are being harassed by a sexually aggressive brother-in-law (an all-too-common scenario) or sister-in-law? You feel caught in a double bind. Your loyalty to your spouse's family may prevent you from revealing the unwanted advances. Or, although your own self-respect makes you reluctant to be seen as a victim, you know that if you tell in-laws what is going on, you may be viewed as the instigator.

Sometimes, the incidents will slow down or stop if you avoid being alone with the sexually aggressive sibling-in-law; however, it is my experience that the only way to end the unwanted advances is to let the aggressor know that he or she will be exposed to the entire family if the advances continue. This behavior cannot be tolerated, and I would suggest that it not be kept a family secret, because other members of the family are likely to be experiencing the same behavior.

Let the aggressor know that he or she will be exposed to the entire family.

---

* To protect the privacy of persons mentioned or quoted, names and identifying characteristics have been changed throughout the book.

5. *Send your pregnant sister-in-law an article that discusses birth defects.*

Like the in-laws who constantly offer unsolicited advice, insensitive siblings-in-law can wreak havoc on an unsuspecting newcomer to the family. It seems that each family has its share of know-it-alls, those experts on everything, who insist on giving you solutions to what they consider all of *your* life's problems.

Do You See Yourself?

If you have developed some of these horrible in-law patterns, it is not too late to turn them around and try to make a change. Changing yourself may not change your in-laws, but it may make you feel better about your in-law relationship.

Sometimes, we forget that in-laws are people too. They actually did have a childhood. They do have hopes and dreams, and they do like to play and have fun, just as much as we do. They like to have friends in and may be romantically involved in relationships with others. Fun is not restricted to the territory of children.

People generally do make compromises in life for the people they love and care about.

Think about what type of in-law you are and want to be, and realize that people generally do make compromises in life for the people they love and care about. Rather than trying to keep your in-laws out of your family, explore how to include them in constructive and positive ways. For this to happen, you must respect and honor your in-law's territory, as well as your own.

The Good Parent-in-Law

Give advice only when asked.

When you are not aware of the impact of your behavior on others, you risk ruining a new in-law relationship. Being what you consider a "good enough" parent-in-law is a challenge. You are not only judged by yourself and your family but also by the standards of society. Historically, much has been expected from parents-in-law, especially mothers-in-law. Making the move from being a responsible parent to being an in-law is tricky. The little things that you said prior to your child's marriage, such as "Don't forget to take an umbrella," or "Let us know what time you will be back," suddenly are seen as an invasion of privacy rather than the comments of a concerned, caring parent. A positive shift for parents-in-law is to give advice only when asked and to support the development of the next generation and the right of its members to learn from their own mistakes. A sense of humor and a long-view perspective are valuable assets to parents-in-law as they negotiate this most interesting stage of life.

Parents-in-Law as Experienced Advisers

When clients' children are getting married, I suggest that the parents see themselves as *experienced advisers* to married children rather than *parents* of married children. If you are facing a role as a parent-in-law, you need to be aware that, although you may have expertise, you do not have the authority to make things happen. For example, remembering your struggles to go through college while supporting a wife and two young children, you may wish that your new son-in-law would finish his college degree before the couple begins a family. But because you are dealing with other adults, you must realize that your advice will be seen only as a suggestion, and will often not carry much weight. On the other hand, although you may not have the final say on some issues, you should not discount the amount of influence that you do have as a parent-in-law.

Realize that your advice will be seen only as a suggestion.

To be viewed as an experienced adviser, you need to believe in yourself. The answers are not "out there somewhere;" they are actually within you. Because of your past experience with your own in-laws, you have an idea of what an in-law should be, and sometimes these roles can be accepted without exploring how they might be changed.

The Good Child-in-Law

It is interesting to contemplate the differences between being a child-in-law and a parent-in-law, especially in light of the fact that both the children-in-law and the parents-in-law are (usually) legally adults. However, each is in a different place in terms of life cycle and life experiences.

"Why," you might ask yourself, "do specific in-laws not like or understand me?" Or, "Why do I not like or understand them?" To get answers, step back and take a look at your personal contribution to the relationship.

You have looked at in-law types. Now take a slightly different perspective and look at in-law needs.

There is nothing right or wrong about these needs.

The key to child-in-law and parent-in-law friction may lie in differing needs. In their work with in-laws, Linda Berg-Cross and Jacqueline Jackson have identified five personality variables as those that most affect in-law relationships: (1) Control, (2) Inclusion, (3) Intimacy, (4) Problem Solving, and (5) Helping Behaviors. There is nothing right or wrong about these needs, and looking at them can give insight into our own and others' points of view. The following personality needs, along with typical in-law comments, will give you an idea of the differences in in-law perspectives. Read them over and then rate *your* needs as compared to your in-laws' needs.

Control Needs

Some individuals have a high need to control decisions and activities in their lives. This need for control is often a defense against a fear of being out of control.

FATHER-IN-LAW: "It drives me nuts when people don't make plans. I like to have everything nailed down, including what and where we will eat."

Or, in order to feel in control, these people will change something about the plan.

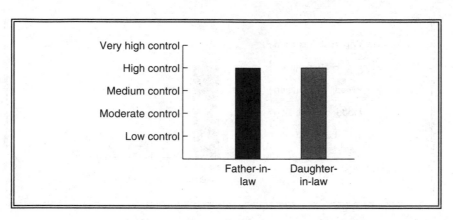

Control Needs

DAUGHTER-IN-LAW: "Why don't we meet at 10:00 rather than 10:30? I'll drive. Let's take a lunch rather than buy."

Inclusion Needs

For some in-laws, it is important to be included in shared times and important events; for others, it is not. In-laws who have a high inclusion need (the need to be liked or loved, and to be part of the lives of their loved ones) have great difficulty understanding those with a low inclusion need.

In-laws who have a high inclusion need have great difficulty understanding those with a low inclusion need.

SISTER-IN-LAW: (high inclusion) "She didn't ask me to be her bridesmaid. They went on vacation without us. They never invite us to dinner. I invite them to all the children's school events, but they never come."

SON-IN-LAW: (low inclusion) "I don't want to play games with my in-laws. Why do we have to go to dinner every Sunday anyway? On the weekends, I need some downtime."

How do your inclusion needs compare? Do you feel shut out? Or are you shutting out your in-laws because you have low inclusion needs and they have high inclusion needs?

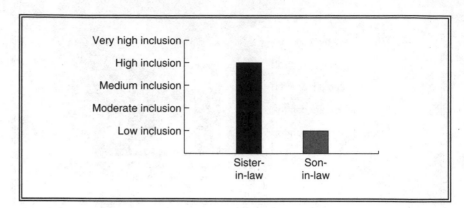

Scale of Inclusion

Intimacy Needs

These are each individual's need for touching, hugging, kissing, and other expressions of intense relationships.

MOTHER-IN-LAW: (high intimacy needs) "He seems so distant. He never wants to touch."

BROTHER-IN-LAW: (low intimacy needs) "My in-laws are always kissing and hugging and then they're slapping or pinching my fanny. A handshake is just fine with me."

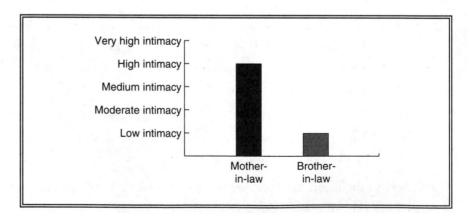

Scale of Intimacy

If an in-law has low intimacy needs and yours are high, maybe you should not take what feels like a cold shoulder or a turned cheek so personally. Some in-laws may not need or want hugs and kisses.

Problem-Solving Needs

We all have learned behaviors for dealing with problems and decisions. We tend to repeat them over and over. Situations change, but our coping repertoire remains limited: "I can tell you right now how my in-law will act." In-law problem-solving behaviors include aggressive, assertive, compliant, or withdrawal styles. Here are some examples.

Situations change, but our coping repertoire remains limited.

SISTER-IN-LAW: (aggressive) "I'm taking my children to the wedding reception whether they were invited or not."

FATHER-IN-LAW: (assertive) "I wish he would speak up. I never know what he is thinking."

MOTHER-IN-LAW: (compliant) "I don't mind if you use my ticket to see *Phantom of the Opera* without me. I'll stay home and babysit."

SON-IN-LAW: (withdrawal) "When he talks in that loud voice, I just space out."

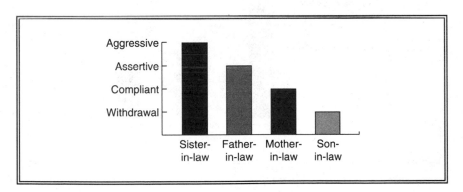

Problem-Solving Needs

Do you think that your style of problem solving is complementary with the style of your parents-in-law, or might it cause friction? Are you or your in-laws high on the scale (aggressive) or low (withdrawal)? If you are at a compliant or withdrawal level, you need to move toward being more assertive. Withdrawal is not the answer, and compliant in-laws often get used as door mats.

Helping Behaviors

You and your in-laws have expectations of appropriate helping behaviors for each generation.

DAUGHTER-IN-LAW: (capable of asking) "I wish she wouldn't empty the dishwasher and offer to run the vacuum every time she visits. If I want help, I'll ask for help."

MOTHER-IN-LAW: (chronic helper) "I think it is important to pitch in and help. I don't want to be seen as a slacker."

FATHER-IN-LAW: (resentful helper) "I wish that my son-in-law wouldn't try to get me to change the oil in the car every time I come to visit. He just can't sit still."

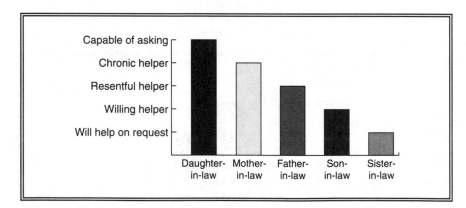

Helping Behaviors

SON-IN-LAW: (willing helper) "You guys are moving this weekend? I'll bring my truck and lend a hand."

SISTER-IN-LAW: (will help on request) "I am more than willing to babysit for my sister and brother-in-law, as long as I have two weeks' notice."

It is too easy to assume that others have our same needs and opinions. If an in-law has a need for inclusion, you might try a simple intervention such as calling your in-law on a weekly basis. Or, buy a box of note cards, and pop one in the mail to your in-law on a regular basis, just to say "hello." Realize that if you want space, or inclusion, you must let your in-laws know.

If you want space, or inclusion, you must let your in-laws know.

These variables should help you to identify, observe, and differentiate your own individual style of behavior and encourage observations on how meeting your own needs can infringe on the needs of other family members.

The Good Sibling-in-Law

Many people are so caught up in the parent-in-law/child-in-law situation that sibling-in-law relationships, which can range from rewarding to uneventful to problematic, are often overlooked. Individuals or couples seldom come to therapy to deal directly with a sibling-in-law problem; however, therapists hear of them often, especially where financial issues and family businesses are concerned. Sibling-in-law problems are most likely not a major issue in therapy because these problems are generally avoided, ignored, or overshadowed by the more dramatic parent-in-law/child-in-law problems.

A sibling-in-law relationship can be termed a *referent relationship* because, in most cases, a relationship with one's in-laws exists only in relationship to one's spouse. However, sometimes in-laws have been part of the same crowd or have introduced their sibling to the future spouse. Hence, siblings-in-law sometimes enter the relationship with a past history that may or may not be amicable.

A relationship that you and your siblings had with your siblings-in-law prior to marriage is echoed in your current family relationships.

You may not think that your partner's brothers and sisters are an important factor in your life. However, you may find that a relationship that you and your siblings had with your siblings-in-law prior to marriage is echoed in your current family relationships. If you were used by your partner during the dating period to pull him or her out of the family soup, there may be a physical or emotional cutoff that will not be welcomed by other family members. On the other hand, your siblings-in-law can be used as scapegoats by your partner, in dealing with your unresolved problems as a couple. I have heard many sisters and brothers blame the spouse of their sibling (their sibling-in-law) when they have little or no contact with their beloved brother or sister (who, if the truth were known, is often happy not to have family contact). Despite their potential to bring conflict to a family, siblings-in-law can also be a source of fun and entertainment. Because they usually share a close age proximity, many siblings-in-law have common outlooks on politics, music, and entertainment. And because they are peers, siblings-in-law can become good friends—or mortal enemies.

Stop for a moment and think about your expectations toward your siblings-in-law. What kind of a sibling-in-law would you like to be? What kind of a sibling-in-law have you been? What would you like your future to be as a sibling-in-law? Have you had some past difficult relationships with your siblings-in-law? They do not have to continue into the future.

Take these things in stride and forgive and live and let live.

Often, older siblings-in-law may have been or are critical of the younger brothers and sisters and their partners. They may deliver some harsh criticisms about siblings-in-law who are going through their teenage years. If you have been a target of these criticisms, you can learn, as you become an adult, to take these things in stride and forgive and live and let live.

A client, Nancy, told me that her sister-in-law, her oldest brother's wife, had been very critical of her when she was a teenager. Nancy dressed with the times, wearing short skirts and scoop-necked dresses. Her sister-in-law would say that she should not be dressing that way or she should not be going out that late. The older sister-in-law let everyone know that she felt her younger sister-in-law was flighty and promiscuous. Later on, when Nancy married and had her own children, she dealt with her sister-in-law on a formal basis and was willing to get together with her at family outings and to treat her civilly, but she never felt very close.

Birth Order

Is it nature or nurture? Now that you have looked at your personality type and needs, take a look at your birth order and at your sibling-in-law's birth order. You may find a key to some of your problems. Dr. Kevin Leman, in *The Birth Order Book*, states that birth order has powerful influences on your entire life. According to Dr. Leman, some of the most compatible marriages are made when the oldest child from one family marries the youngest child from another. If you or your sibling marry the most compatible child in a family in terms of birth order, logic says that you may not be compatible with your spouse's siblings. Looking at birth order can be another aspect of helping you to assess yourself as well as your in-laws.

Now is the time to look at your attitude and to make a change if you think that an in-law relationship might be worth salvaging. Do you want to enjoy more closeness and more commonality, since you are both involved with the same man or woman as partner or sibling? If for no other reason, be civil with your siblings-in-law because you *will* be getting together during times of crises—divorce, death of a partner, a parent, or a child, and, sometimes, family business matters. On the other hand, you can choose to be a terrible sibling-in-law.

Look at your attitude and make a change if you think that an in-law relationship might be worth salvaging.

Can People Change?

Changing your in-law relationships may take energy as well as nerve. You may ask yourself, "What if my in-laws do not like me?" or "What if they do not want to see me anymore?" Can not having your in-laws see you be worse than seeing them under the difficult circumstances you are currently experiencing?

At first, you probably will get it wrong and you may say the wrong thing.

"What if I get it wrong?" At first, you probably will get it wrong and you may say the wrong thing. But what goes around comes around, and you will probably have a chance to apologize or to correct what you have said the next time the same topic comes up in conversation.

If you find yourself in an unlivable in-law relationship, you may decide to take action that could end the relationship. Are you willing to pay that price? Sometimes, the need for change makes it worth the risk of a permanent cutoff, especially if the situation does have a possibility for improvement. It is sometimes helpful to take a worst-case-scenario approach: "The worst that could happen if I say something is that my in-law will avoid me." However, I believe that, with sufficient desire, change is positive and we can turn negative situations around.

Take Your In-Law Temperature

Think back to the in-law personality types, needs, and birth order described earlier. While considering these, determine where you are and where would like to be on an in-law thermometer.

Loving. "I couldn't have asked for a better in-law. I'm glad you married my family member."

Generous. "We know that these early years are tough, and want you to know that we've set aside some money for each of our children, to help out when you buy your first house."

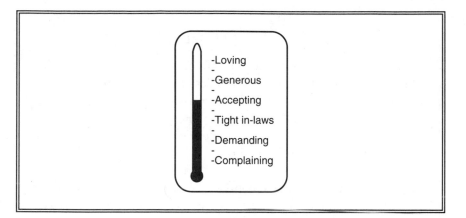

In-Law Thermometer

Accepting. "I'm so pleased that my child found such a wonderful person. I'm sure they will be very happy and the new spouse will be a nice addition to our family."

Tight In-Laws. "I want to spend time with the kids as long as they contribute what I consider is their fair share. I put in a lot of hard work to make myself financially secure. Now they should do the same thing."

Demanding. "I feel that my parents-in-law should spend holidays and vacations with us. I also expect weekly letters and daily phone check-ins."

Complaining. "I want the children to come, but I don't care for the extra work and noise . . . if only they would pitch in."

Worksheet

Now that you have taken your in-law temperature and explored your other in-law qualities, stop and think for a moment about the changes you can make to stay in your in-law comfort zone. Following are five recommendations for keeping a temperate in-law climate. Start with the one that seems easiest to you. After you have mastered that, move on to another.

1. Refuse to take pot shots at in-laws or engage in in-law bashing. Stay neutral. If an in-law does something that irritates you, try to describe objectively how the behavior or situation makes you feel: "When you . . . , I feel . . . ."

2. Give advice sparingly and remember the best in-law advice is no advice. Express your reaction to the in-law's behavior or the situation in a nonjudgmental way. "I feel . . . ."

3. Maintain your sense of humor. In-laws do say the funniest things. Be willing to laugh with in-laws and to see yourself through their eyes.

4. Negotiate in-law differences. These are, after all, long-term relationships. If you feel comfortable asking for change, specify one or two behavior changes: "I would prefer . . ."; "I want . . ."; "I would like . . . ."

5. Give your in-laws the benefit of a doubt, and hope they will do the same for you. If your in-laws do something you just cannot tolerate, offer alternatives. No one likes having to capitulate to demands. "Would you rather . . . or . . . ?"

PART TWO

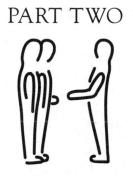

STAGES OF THE
IN-LAW RELATIONSHIP

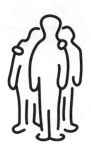

Norming,

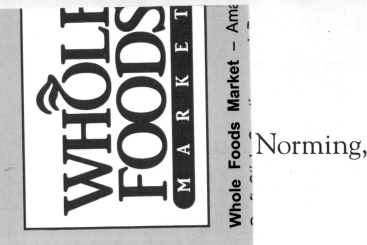

-law relationship needs to be ne-
tarting with integrating a new

r family. How do you and mem-
hily member? Are you open and
w members to prove themselves?
-law? Is there any correlation be-
w and how you treat others com-

Most of us do not recognize the subtle but dramatic changes in societal expectations that occur with a new marriage. These changes in status create corresponding requirements for changed behavior. As we move through the cycles of our relationships, there are predictable—as well as unpredictable—stages that we must work through in order for our in-law relationships to thrive.

Our natural progression through the life stages may bring some surprises for future parents- and children-in-law, who often say, "We got along so well before the wedding and then there was a big change." Virginia Satir, a pioneering family therapist, describes the phenomenon of the *pseudo-self*, the pleasant, amicable person we project to casual acquaintances. The *face* we present to those whom we infrequently meet can become fatiguing when it must be assumed over the long haul. But no in-laws can be on their *company best* at all times, and as in-laws get to know each

*There are
predictable stages
in in-law
relationships.*

other better, care must be taken that all parties feel relaxed enough to show their true selves—the disagreeable along with the charming. Only with true mutual acceptance of the other can this relaxation occur, and, paradoxically, only when people can relax with each other (thus being free to show their occasional unattractive attributes) can true friendship—or kinship—develop.

News of Difference—What In-Laws Grow Up With

A new person coming into the family brings the news of difference.

Bringing a new person into the family can create a certain amount of dissension, contention, or even amusement, because the person coming into the family brings what Gregory Bateson termed *the news of difference.*

A person new to the family introduces a different point of view and a different focus on issues. This perspective can be surprising to the rest of the family, because they are used to their family's rules and norms about what is and is not discussed.

People think that what they have grown up with is normal. When an in-law comes into their family, they may point out the "odd" behaviors that their new family member displays. On either side, there may be a history of destructive behaviors—physical or verbal abuse, or alcoholism; or petty peculiarities that family members have long grown accustomed to; or serious problems. Criticism of these behaviors, especially in public, can lead to the distancing of a new in-law.

A Fresh Point of View

Rather than declaring the new in-law a problem, welcome the in-law as a newcomer who has a fresh point of view and different ideas that will broaden and enrich the family.

As humans, we are more alike than we are different and we tend to marry people from similar backgrounds; therefore, most ideas that are brought into a family are not going to be too far afield from the ideals already held and cherished. However, if new in-laws adhere to large cultural or religious differences, it may be difficult to accept their viewpoints. Family members, as well as the new in-laws, may want to wait and watch and observe rather than rush into judgment or make pronouncements that may end up in an alienating standoff.

Try looking at in-laws as another ingredient to enrich the family stew and to make life a little more interesting and spicy.

Stages of In-Law Relationships

Most in-law relationships develop in predictable stages, as identified for small groups by Bruce Tuckman. The in-law stages are:

Stage	In-Law Task
Forming	Meeting the clan
Storming	Learning the rules of the house/shaking out
Norming	Settling in and agreeing to disagree
Conforming	Being seen (and feeling) a part of the clan

Each stage brings its own milestones and tasks—and each stage is a normal and necessary part of cultivating a healthy in-law relationship. It is best not to rush through the stages. You will have a lifetime to work on your in-law relationships.

Forming: Meeting the Clan

The first stage is the getting acquainted or *forming* stage. This develops during the dating period, when there are introductions to parents,

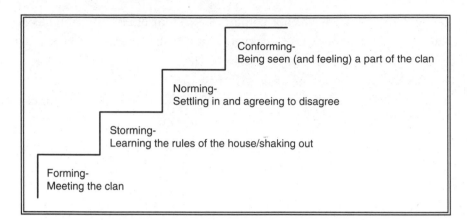

Conforming-
Being seen (and feeling) a part of the clan

Norming-
Settling in and agreeing to disagree

Storming-
Learning the rules of the house/shaking out

Forming-
Meeting the clan

Stages of Meeting In-Laws

The first stage is the getting acquainted or forming stage.

siblings, and extended family, and invitations to formal and informal family events. During this stage (usually prior to marriage), each person usually puts his or her best foot forward. Only later—when the *pseudo-self* grows weary—do problems surface.

Recognize and honor differences.

One of the principal ways to deal with an in-law relationship in the forming stage is to recognize and honor differences. Rita, a 50-year-old physician, said, "When I met Henry's parents, I wasn't sure about them. I didn't agree with them on religion, politics, or even how to cook a pot roast. I really wasn't even sure if I liked them. But then I had to remember they had raised Henry, and I loved him, so there must be something good about them. At that point, I began to enjoy their differences, and to love them, too."

As your in-law relationships proceed through this initial forming stage, it may be useful for you to think of it as a time of scarce resources, or valuable resources in short supply. We all have a need and a desire to preserve what we may consider our limited resources. Among a family's scarce resources would be tangibles such as money, represented by requests for the family car (the one with the gas tank that always seems to come back empty) or for loans of cash; invitations to dine out; trips; and family outings. Intangible resources such as time, energy, and privacy must also be considered.

Integrating a new member into the family requires a conscious expenditure of all these resources, especially time and energy. For this reason alone, it is important to proceed slowly with getting to know your in-laws. Take the time to identify their likes and dislikes and to get to know them as real people, and then be willing to expend the energy and time needed to work out solutions if there are sensitive areas or differences. One of the primary reasons I see families and individuals at a standstill with in-law problems is that someone gets discouraged and feels that working out the problems is just not worth the investment or effort. This happened to Gladys, one of my clients. She was the second daughter-in-law in the family, and she felt her in-laws had used up all their reserves in welcoming the first daughter-in-law into the family. She tried everything to win them over—fixing meals, cleaning, giving gifts. But they did not respond to any of her overtures. I recommend that if you face these problems, stop trying to win your in-laws over with your actions, and talk directly about the problem. Try to get to know them as people—and give them a chance to know you.

Storming: Learning the Rules/Shaking Out

Following the getting-to-know-you forming stage comes the shaking out, or *storming* stage, when the initial expectations of the in-law relationship change. This may take place after the first year of the relationship and is somewhat determined by how often you see your in-laws. By this stage, the *honeymoon* of the in-law relationship is definitely over and all the little idiosyncrasies and annoyances have been discovered. When they reach this point, many people are fatigued with having to behave at their *company best*. They decide to just be themselves and let it all hang out, warts and all. The mother-in-law, father-in-law, and siblings-in-law who

Next comes the shaking out or storming stage.

were so wonderful during the first year are now found to be imperfect and may even show some annoyance.

Setting Guidelines

Early in a marriage, most encounters between newlyweds and families take place at the home of the parents, thus expanding the potential for numerous uncomfortable in-law situations. The traditional lines of social decorum become muddied in the newly formed relationship. The new member of the family may wonder silently: *What do I do when I need a drink of water? Can I rummage through the refrigerator? Can I open a can of tuna and make a sandwich? Can I help myself to a soda? Do I put the dishes in the dishwasher? Should I expect the in-laws to treat me like a house-guest or like a member of the family? Does the entire family drink out of the glass that is on the sink? Where are the glasses kept, in which cupboard? What is the family's meal schedule? How much do they eat? Am I expected to eat everything on my plate? Should I volunteer to do the dishes? Am I supposed to do the food shopping and cooking next time?*

Bobby's *storming* experience was pretty typical. Two months after their wedding, he and his bride went to his in-laws' cabin on a lake. He stopped in his father-in-law's den and decided to use the computer to write a quick note to his parents. As he was writing, his father-in-law came in and said with an edge to his voice that Bobby could have had the courtesy to ask first, because the computer contained some important data. Bobby said, "This was a side of my father-in-law that I had never seen. He was always polite, congenial, and just a friendly, happy-go-lucky kind of guy while I was dating his daughter. I quickly learned that whenever I used any of his equipment, including his computer or his tools, I needed to first ask, and then replace them very carefully."

Bobby learned a family rule the hard way. The clearer the rules are, the better chance the new in-law has of following them. Most people are not consciously aware of their own family's rules, but you can try to piece together the puzzle by following your spouse's lead. Inevitably, you will make a misstep or break an unwritten law. Apologize, learn, and move on. And remember—the tension of the storming stage is natural.

Redefining Roles

When an in-law is introduced into a family, the entire family must redefine its roles. The son, no longer *our little boy*, takes on adult responsibilities as a husband, lover, and, perhaps, a soon-to-be father. The daughter, no longer *the little princess*, is now a wife, a lover, and perhaps a future mother.

When an in-law is introduced, the entire family must redefine its roles.

The roles and responsibilities of parents-in-law in helping a new union get off to its best start can be challenging. In her study of in-laws, Evelyn R. Duvall identified at least seven roles that are well represented in the behavior of mothers-in-law. These roles can be extended to all in-laws.

Rejecting In-Laws.   By adopting one of these roles, you or your in-laws might show a lack of acceptance for an in-law or potential in-law:

1. **Aggressive opposition:** "My mother always says, 'Tell your husband that dinner is ready and to come to the table,' when he is standing right by her. She refuses to speak directly to him."

2. **Active proselytizing:** "My father-in-law never stops with the work advice. He constantly makes negative comments about my work prospects."

3. **Persistent resistance—a formal politeness:** "My daughter-in-law refuses to call us by our first names even though we have suggested it on several occasions. After a year, she still calls us Mr. Rogers and Mrs. Rogers."

4. **Initial resistance gradually lessening as the marriage continues:** "I thought it would be horrible for my daughter to marry a plumber, but now he's starting to grow on me—I'm impressed with how he treats her and her son from a previous marriage."

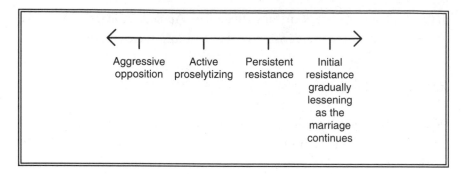

Scale of Resistance-Acceptance

Accepting In-Laws. In these roles, acceptance is the primary factor:

5. **Resigned acceptance:** "I knew they would get married anyway, so I may as well try to like her."

6. **Readiness to explore and accept:** "He seems so nice, and I have to admit that it's so interesting to learn about his Pakistani culture."

7. **Active aid in assimilation:** "Let us know what we can do to help you with your move."

Holding On

Some potential parents-in-law and siblings-in-law may not be ready to have their family member take on the role of husband or wife, thereby abandoning their primary role of child or sibling. In talking about the new couple, Monica McGoldrick says that the new family members (in-laws) are often used as scapegoats to relieve family tension. Indeed, it is less risky to hate one's in-laws than to confront one's own blood relatives. For example, if a son or daughter does not stand up for his or her new spouse, the family may see the spouse as an interloper, and therefore someone whom they can pick on as a low-risk target. The spouse may then become the repository of anger, frustration, and resentment.

Parents and siblings who take this tack risk alienating or losing contact with their blood relative as well as the scapegoated in-law.

Paulinia McCullough writes that if children have established their personality and beliefs separate from their birth family, they have difficulty incorporating their spouses into the family. Indeed, the child may choose a mate who will help him or her fend off the family and who may become a wedge between the mate and the family. Therefore, difficulties you have with your in-laws may be reflections of problems your spouse (or child) had with the family prior to the marriage. By not accepting in-laws into the family, some parents try to continue to hold on to the parent–child role. But holding on too tightly may risk the entire relationship. The hand that holds on should also be able to let go. My client, Richard, an Army officer, wishes he had been more willing to be flexible with his mother-in-law. He said, "My mother-in-law and I fought from day one. She wanted to protect her turf and run her daughter's life, and so did I. My wife ended up dumping both of us."

Negotiating

Person-to-person negotiating can often prevent an irreversible cutoff and bring about an in-law solution. But beware: negotiating is not for the faint of heart. In-laws who want to talk things out must have the heart of a lion, the mind of a lawyer, and the patience of Job. Still, it's worth considering, for the key to successfully navigating the forming and storming stages *can be* negotiation. Try to identify your in-laws' most important issues, then proceed from the most absurd resolution to the most agreeable one.

Negotiation is the key for successfully navigating the forming and storming stages.

One of my clients lamented the fact that her in-laws did not seem to like her two large dogs. I suggested that she let her in-laws know she would be willing to lock up the dogs in a safe area during the times that made the in-laws uncomfortable. She could then ask her in-laws when the dogs were a problem for them. During meals? When they came in the door and the dogs jumped on them? Did her in-laws just not like dogs, or did these large dogs scare them? Did they enjoy the dogs at her house, but prefer not to have them brought to their house? By identifying problem areas, a solution can usually be negotiated.

Negotiation requires a commitment of your time and energy. Prior to embarking on it, you need to ask for an agreement: Are your in-laws interested enough in resolution that they are willing to stay the course? If so, prioritize the areas of disagreement, from easiest-to-resolve to most difficult, and tackle the easiest ones first. Address only one issue during each negotiating session. When the family has prioritized the issues in advance, the issues that are difficult (and often, most important) are dealt with last. This plan theoretically helps the family to move more quickly toward resolution of easier issues, and to gain confidence regarding their ability to resolve more loaded issues.

Yours, Mine, and Ours

Another factor that may be dealt with during the storming or shaking-things-out stage is the involvement of the spouses' in-laws with each other. I sometimes hear clients complain, "I didn't pick him/her or why am I expected to love him/her?" This attitude is often taken a step further when the family is expected to tolerate, or even to love, the parents or siblings of the new in-law.

In some cases, one of the children-in-law or parents-in-law wants both sets of parents to bond in a close relationship. For example, when Jane and David married, Jane felt that her parents and David's parents would naturally be great friends, because she and David had so much in common. Jane put on large dinners and invited both sets of in-laws. She also put pressure on her parents to socialize with David's parents on their own. During the course of therapy, Jane came to realize that her strong need for affiliation was not shared by either set of in-laws. She was putting more energy into the bonding of the families than any of the parents-in-law. To everyone's relief, after several years of trying, Jane gave up on family togetherness and began working on her own relationships with individual family members.

Unless both sets of parents of a new couple have an established relationship prior to the marriage, the idea of joining two extended families generally requires too much logistical energy. A friend comments, "People moving is the hardest work in the world."

Norming: Settling In and Agreeing to Disagree

After families have successfully negotiated the storming or shaking out stage (or, after individuals have run out of energy to keep the conflicts going full-steam), they may begin to move into the *norming* or settling in phase, where boundaries are set or reset, rules are redefined, and members develop an understanding of where each fits within the in-law system. By the second or third year of the marriage, the couple will have begun to move into developing a state of normalcy within the family. Because the individuals now feel comfortable showing their true faces, the in-laws can be used as a dumping ground, an outlet where the couple can safely vent their anger and frustration in their efforts toward trying to adapt to each other. By that time, the in-laws, both parents and children, have come to realize what it means to be an in-law and to try to deal with some of the expectations.

In the norming *stage, boundaries are set and rules are redefined.*

Samuel, a 39-year-old machinist, and his wife Gwen met when they were 15; they were high school sweethearts. At that age, they were pretty callow and did a lot that really annoyed Gwen's parents, who were strict. Gwen ended up being grounded a lot, which led to bitterness and anger on Samuel's part. Ugly things were said, and they all parted on bad terms. "Little did any of us know at the time that, 10 years later, Gwen and I would get back together and marry," said Samuel. "When we got engaged, her family still treated me like an irresponsible teenager, even though a lot of water had passed under the bridge in the meantime. And, to tell you the truth, I did not completely trust them—I fully expected them to cancel the wedding, even up to the point when I saw Gwen walk down the aisle on her dad's arm." It has been said that time heals all wounds; within a few years, Gwen's family realized that Samuel had grown up.

Moving into Adulthood

As you can see from Samuel's narrative, negotiating the norming stage requires being somewhat philosophical. Samuel seemed to have put the past into some kind of perspective. He was willing to give Gwen's family time to realize that he was no longer an irresponsible teenager and had become a competent adult. I believe this is one purpose of the marriage ceremony: to help families to begin to move from the shaking out of the storming stage toward the norming stage. A ritual marriage ceremony helps parents-in-law (who earlier had recited the same or similar vows) to recognize and accept the fact that the couple is moving into adulthood.

Forgiveness Rituals

Some actions and sentiments expressed while limits are being developed in the storming stage may leave bruises or open wounds. If this is the case and your in-law family has not regained a state of normalcy, family members may need to go through a process of forgiveness toward the parents-in-law and the children-in-law. Simple rituals may help with this process.

Rituals of forgiveness can include happy family events.

Family events can be used as rituals. Give a son-in-law with whom you have been angry a surprise birthday party; or take your daughter-in-law to lunch and a fashion show. Inviting in-laws over for a candlelight dinner is a nice way to display your responsibility as well as your caring toward in-laws.

Rituals can also be more elaborate: One couple took their children and *their* spouses to Hawaii, where the parental couple had a renewal of vows. They invited their estranged son-in-law and daughter to take part in the ceremony. The ritual was conducted by a priest on a beautiful beach, and both couples reported that it was a very healing event. They renewed not only their vows but the kinship and friendship aspects of the biological family and the family-through-marriage.

With improved relationships, your family can move forward in the norming stage. In the best outcome, the majority of in-laws will develop a cordial, warm, and loving relationship with you.

Rules? What Rules?

Defining expectations and rules is an important step during the norming phase. Settling in and boundaries may need to be set by the biological child or parent in order to protect the in-law who brings in new skills. Kitty and Jeff confronted the boundary issue. Early in the marriage, Kitty's parents frequently asked Jeff to help out with home repairs. As a new son-in-law, Jeff felt obligated to help, but resented the demands. Matters came to a head when Kitty's mom and dad just assumed Jeff would be willing to spend his vacation helping them fix up their cabin. Kitty confronted her parents about this and, after a year, told her parents to stop asking Jeff to help them. The parents-in-law were chagrined, but were willing to reframe the relationship and were pleased when Jeff offered to help out with odd jobs.

Anyone stepping into a new in-law family quickly discovers that things are not always as they seem. A new in-law may think that the father- or mother-in-law is making the major family decisions, but, after looking at the situation, may find that one or the other seems to manipulate the outcome the majority of the time. It benefits the new in-law to understand the age and authority hierarchies of the in-law family and to

Understand the age and authority hierarchies of the in-law family.

understand who is *most* in charge, and will be making the key decisions. Some decision making is not the prerogative of the parents. For example, Miguel came to therapy and told me that although his father-in-law was quite stern, he did not necessarily rule the roost. Shortly after his wedding, Miguel realized that his wife's oldest sister, who lived with the parents, was really the boss. "It is very subtle, but everyone in the family defers to her desires," said Miguel. "My wife once invited her folks to come over for lunch and they said, 'We'll check with Paula and let you know.'" Miguel noted that nobody in his wife's family saw what was going on. Sisters-in-law beware: My research shows that where there are in-law problems in the family, sisters-in-law score second to mothers-in-law as most problematic.

Once you discover who is *really* in charge, you can learn to work *with*, rather than *against*, that person. In the beginning of an in-law relationship, I suggest that you respect the existing structure and let a little time pass before you decide to rock the boat. Remember, your relationship with your spouse has connections with your in-laws' family structure. If changes are to be made, they must be made in the context of that marriage structure, whether you rebel or go with the flow. For example, if the oldest sister usually plans all the family events and the new brother-in-law wants to put together a day at the horse races, he might consider using her as a sounding board, getting her consensus, and even letting her work out all the details. In this way, the siblings-in-law can get to know each other, test the waters, and learn to work within the existing family system.

When various roles are clarified and accepted, family members can develop mutual respect for one another. In-laws will then feel comfortable collaborating on the decision-making process or even suggesting changes.

From working cooperatively, a team spirit is built and strong roots for a new kinship are formed. Realigned loyalties and mutual respect allow in-laws the freedom to really be themselves. Rather than causing conflict, differences can be respected, negotiated, or ignored.

Conforming: Being Seen as Part of the Clan

If your in-law family successfully completes the forming, storming, and norming stages, *conforming* is where maximum cohesion is reached. Most rules and bonds, both implicit and explicit, have been established and accepted. Where they have not been established, there is a tolerable amount of static. Minimal social and emotional expectations have been met, and you and your in-laws have at least laid the foundation to negotiate future problems, conflicts, or misunderstandings. Once they have reached this stage, the children-in-law and parents-in-law have learned more about give and take and have reached some level of agreement in their mutual expectations.

In the conforming stage, maximum cohesion is reached.

You Are Never Home Free

Although you may feel that you and your in-laws have essentially achieved a conforming relationship during the early relationship period and that you have a solid foundation for dealing with future problems, remember that the family is subject to many outside forces. Changes, especially the life cycle changes of birth, divorce, retirement, and death, will shake the family. (This area is explored in depth in Chapter 6.) Your knowledge of such changes, and your understanding and expectation that flexibility is constantly needed, will help you and your in-laws to preserve your bond through the ups and downs of extended family life.

Think of your extended family as a boat moving along a river, and think of yourself as a water skier riding behind it. If the family boat has a crisis or lifestyle change or the river has an unexpected turn, the in-laws will need to adjust the boat's course. The family boat is subject to waves and wakes, and sometimes you may just have to hang on, keep your balance, and try not to make the wrong moves.

Negotiating the Stages Throughout the Relationship: An Ongoing Cycle

Be aware that the constellations of feelings and activities in any given stage, such as forming or storming, do not occur in a linear fashion. You may be in a norming relationship with one in-law and in a constant storming stage with another.

Assess what stage you are in with each in-law.

The questions for you may well be:

- "Where am I with each in-law?"

- "Am I moving through these stages, or am I stuck in a certain stage with a particular in-law?"

Target Relationships

One of my client couples decided to target the wife's father-in-law as an in-law relationship that they would like to work on. Jen said, "my father-in-law is a real jerk and has been since day one." She saw her relationship with him as still being in the storming stage. In fact, she said that if she were in a workplace with him, she would sue him for sexual harassment because he constantly told sexist jokes and tried to kiss her on the lips.

She decided that, to deal with her father-in-law in this storming stage, she would have to tell him, in as kind a way as possible, how she felt about his sexist comments. Otherwise, they could never move into the norming stage, because she was not willing to let these sexually inappropriate remarks be part of her relationship with him. Jen decided she would start out with his kissing behavior. In the past, whenever she visited his house, he grabbed her and gave her a big mushy kiss. The next time she arrived at the house and her father-in-law tried to give her a kiss, she put her arm out and said, "I think it would be more appropriate if we shook hands." At first, the father-in-law was a bit shocked and offended at her assertiveness, but he accepted the offer of a friendly handshake.

Jen reported that things improved from there. When he tried to get closer to her or to make comments, she would just say that it was not appropriate. She started to set a limit with her father-in-law, which, several years later, she found useful when the couple had children and she wanted to set other limits with him. She says her father-in-law continues to be overbearing but he now realizes that she has her limits and is not willing to have him step over the line. She believes he respects her for this behavior, and she knows it will be a good example for her daughter and son. Their norming has turned into respect for Jen's rights as a woman and a mother and for her boundaries as a person.

Throughout your relationship, you and your in-laws will continue to encounter the issues of each of these stages, as life-cycle changes bring new circumstances to the family. Learning to accept and even love one's in-laws is a process that comes through a lifetime of experiences.

Stages of In-Law Relationships—Overview

Just as medical patients find it beneficial to have their illnesses given a definite diagnosis, many individuals and families in therapy find it helpful to identify the stages they are encountering in the in-law relationship. Below are some questions that may help you to determine how the members of your family are processing the issues, and to identify areas where there is a risk of getting stuck in any given stage.

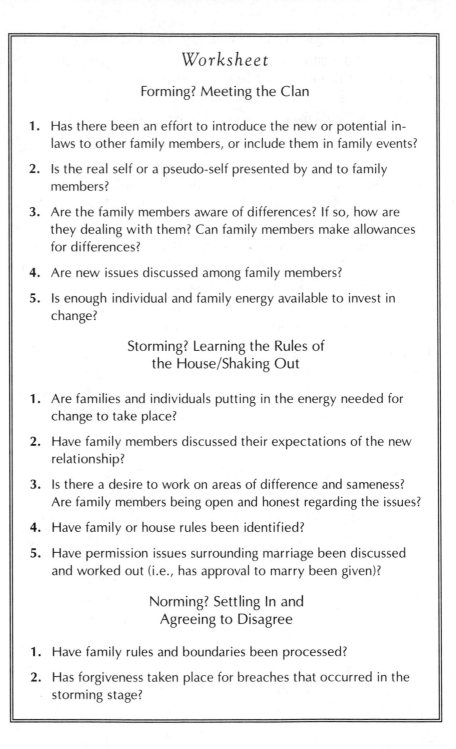

Worksheet

Forming? Meeting the Clan

1. Has there been an effort to introduce the new or potential in-laws to other family members, or include them in family events?

2. Is the real self or a pseudo-self presented by and to family members?

3. Are the family members aware of differences? If so, how are they dealing with them? Can family members make allowances for differences?

4. Are new issues discussed among family members?

5. Is enough individual and family energy available to invest in change?

Storming? Learning the Rules of the House/Shaking Out

1. Are families and individuals putting in the energy needed for change to take place?

2. Have family members discussed their expectations of the new relationship?

3. Is there a desire to work on areas of difference and sameness? Are family members being open and honest regarding the issues?

4. Have family or house rules been identified?

5. Have permission issues surrounding marriage been discussed and worked out (i.e., has approval to marry been given)?

Norming? Settling In and Agreeing to Disagree

1. Have family rules and boundaries been processed?

2. Has forgiveness taken place for breaches that occurred in the storming stage?

Worksheet
(Continued)

3. Have individual and family differences been acknowledged and respected?

4. Are the family roles defined and aligned?

5. Do newcomers to the family understand where the power lies? Can a balance of power be reached?

6. Can family members agree to disagree and live with ambiguity and differences? Is it recognized that all issues will not be resolved?

7. Are global issues, such as whether parents share a part of the children's lives, recognized as being more important than one person's being right on any given issue?

Conforming? Being Seen (and Feeling) a Part of the Clan

1. Is the family moving in the same direction and accepting differences?

2. Has the family made accommodations for new issues and individuals coming into the system?

3. Is there love at home? Can people achieve their goals in a nurturing environment?

4. Does the family structure promote the well-being of individual family members?

5. Has equilibrium been reached, that is, do family members express a tolerable level of comfort with the state of the family?

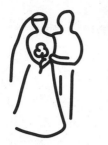

4

Marrying the Family

We Fall in Love and Walk into Marriage— Why We Choose Our Mates

How is the choice of spouse made?

Given the many factors that can cause marital and in-law discord, it is amazing any of us marry at all. How is the choice of spouse made? Although some experts feel that choice of mate is random, others observe that mate selection is most often made for a very strong reason, although the motivation may not be on a conscious level. When you married, you may have been looking for what Arthur L. Leader calls *proper in-laws*—those who meet your expectations of what an in-law should be. Or you may have been attracted to in-laws who are either just like your family or very different from your family. In previous chapters we have looked at personality issues and needs that affect your in-law relationships. Here are some in-law configurations you may have sought, or unwittingly ended up joining to satisfy your personal needs:

In-Law Characteristics

- **Happy-family in-laws:** In-laws who share your vision of the family as a happy, pleasant group.

- **Touchy-feely in-laws:** In-laws who will provide the love and support you felt you missed while growing up.

- **Status in-laws (marrying up):** In-laws who have higher social status and can possibly provide some financial support.

- **Nonsupportive in-laws:** In-laws who continue to validate that the world is hard and cruel and who reflect past negative experiences in relationships.

Your Personal Needs

- **To make a connection:** You sought a feeling of community with a unit or force larger than yourself, to provide you with continuity and belonging.

- **To take on a project:** Your in-law family has problems and you want to help your partner work them out; or, you are acting out your own family-of-origin issues. In the past, you may have felt powerless. Now you feel strong and needed, because marriage to the right mate lets you feel powerful in the family arena.

- **To replace lost family members:** Your in-laws take the place of family members who have been lost through divorce or death. Someone who has suffered the death of a beloved family member often marries into a nurturing family.

Permission to Marry

During therapy sessions, I frequently open the discussion by asking couples in crisis whether they thought their parents approved of their marriage. They often reply, "Isn't it a bit old-fashioned to think that a couple needs to get permission or approval from their parents to marry?" It may seem out-of-date, but I believe that marriages should start out with as much going for them as possible, and getting parental blessings by asking for approval to marry is one aspect that is often overlooked. I have discovered that a common thread running through many troubled marriages is that the parents did not give permission or approval and were

Parental blessings can help ward off problems.

therefore not supportive of the marriage or of the potential in-law. I hear statements like, "We told them they were too young," "I told them they weren't ready," "We never wanted them to get married," or, "I warned her not to." Do these sound familiar to you? Did a relationship break up because your significant other's family did not approve of you? Are you an in-law who has withheld approval and security or overtly wants the in-law or interloper out of the family?

M. Duncan Stanton of the University of Rochester Medical Center Family Therapy Training Program postulates that, among failed marriages, 80 percent of the couples had not received permission to succeed in the marriage. According to Stanton, this lack of permission originates with the parents. If you are still in the dating stage and considering marriage, you might want to have a discussion with your future mate about asking both sets of parents for their child's hand in marriage.

As a parent-in-law or as a potential child-in-law, ask yourself these questions:

	Parents-In-Law Questions	*Children-In-Law Questions*
Premarital Questions	Am I giving my child's friend the respect I would give a future in-law?	Am I treating my partner's parents in a way that I would want to treat my future in-laws?
	Is it important that my children ask for permission to marry?	Is getting my in-laws' approval to marry their child important to me?
Marital Question	Have I given my child permission to be married to the person he/she has married?	Do I feel that I have my parent-in-law's permission to be married to his or her child?

Asking for permission to marry or live together may help a young couple to work out difficulties with future in-laws prior to the formal or legal beginnings of the relationship—while they are still pre-in-laws. If the future in-laws refuse to give their approval, at least the couple knows where they stand. Differences can then be brought into the open.

If you are a mother- or father-in-law who has never given approval to an in-law, you might want to think about moving in the direction of giving approval. You may have to do it very directly. If the gap between you has been painful, approach the daughter- or son-in-law of whom you initially did not approve.

Prior to the 20th century, parents in America were expected to assume real responsibility for their children's mate selection and courtship behavior, and for the marriage itself. This is no longer the case; however, some very traditional fathers still dare to ask, "What are your intentions, young man?" I know this is true, because such a father lives in my own home (my husband Phil), and our three sons-in-law have survived the question.

Withholding Approval to Marry

Research and common sense suggest that parents think seriously *before* withholding support to a couple who are contemplating marriage. Researchers and family therapists have found that when marriage compatibility tests are taken by young couples, all but a few of the couples get married regardless of the results of the compatibility testing. Over time, close to 80 percent of couples who scored in the incompatible range become divorced. This shows that couples will marry over all objections and, in fact, that objections often strengthen their resolve to marry. But take heart. Change of attitude can make a difference, as seen in the following case.

Clay and Deborah came to therapy because they had experienced a stormy marriage for five years, and, although they loved one another, they were considering divorce. Clay said that none of this was a surprise; prior to their marriage, all of their friends and future in-laws had told them they were not suited for one another. Rather than discouraging them from marrying each other, these dismal prognostications only encouraged them. Clay told me that his mother-in-law went so far as to make appointments for psychological testing, at which time the therapist said that the tests showed them to be highly incompatible. Now, five years and three small children later, they came to me discouraged and resigned to the fact that their parents and friends had been correct—their marriage was indeed doomed.

After several individual sessions in which we discussed their differing styles, we had a session with Deborah's parents. During the course of therapy, the premarital psychological testing was mentioned, and Deborah's mother laughed with embarrassment and told us, "We all took those tests." She then said that Clay was a "wonderful son-in-law and husband" and that, as parents, they would do everything in their power to help the couple work out their relationship. Thus, after five years and lots of conflict, the mother finally granted marital permission. The point here is that couples marry for reasons other than compatibility. If parents-in-law want to support their children in marriage, they need to realize that marriage was the couple's decision to make, and acceptance can have an important impact on the success (or failure) of the marriage. I recently spoke to Clay and Deborah. They continue to work on their marriage, and Clay has pursued individual counseling to work on family-of-origin issues.

What Have You Got to Lose?

Some parents-in-law will not agree to give permission to the marriage. For example, Roxanne, my client, was a single mother with one adult son, Kevin. She was annoyed that Kevin had eloped with Regina, whom she did not meet until after the honeymoon. Roxanne could never forgive her daughter-in-law, Regina, for "stealing" Kevin from her, and, after more than 12 years, continued to harbor a lot of anger and bitterness.

Because the couple was living on the opposite coast, I suggested to Roxanne that she act out what she *would* say if Kevin and Regina were in my office. I had her sit across from an empty chair in which she imagined Regina sitting. Roxanne proceeded to tell Regina how she felt and then she moved into the chair and answered as Regina. After a few sessions, Roxanne realized that Regina had not stolen Kevin from her; Kevin had left, of his own accord, many years earlier. Once she got beyond the bitterness, she was able to welcome Regina into the family and reestablish a better relationship with the couple. You may want to try this technique, too, if you have something you would like to say to an in-law but have no opportunity (or desire) for a face-to-face meeting.

Factors Affecting In-Laws' Approval or Disapproval of Choice of Spouse

Most parents want to share the benefit of their experiences with their children, to help them make a better life and have better marriages than they had. Parents also must be aware that trying to help their children avoid the wrong marriage can be a method of reliving their fondest fantasies, past mistakes, and disappointments in how their own lives have turned out.

The issues affecting choice of spouse and approval of the new family member by parents-in-law are related to age, education, and socioeconomic status, as well as religious, cultural, and ethnic variables.

Age

Many parents feel that their children are not old enough to get married. This sometimes seems to be related to the age of the parents when they were married, and usually arises when the children are on the younger end of the age spectrum. I often hear comments like, "I was too young

Many parents feel that their children are not old enough to get married.

when I got married; I should have listened to my parents," or "Had I known what I know today, I would not have gotten married so early."

There are no hard-and-fast rules about ideal age differentials between spouses; however, we do know that marriages stand a better chance of success when there are common interests. Parents-in-law should be concerned when the bride is extremely young—including under legal age—and the groom seems to be coercive, pushing the young woman into a marriage. But consider the consequences if you withhold consent and the marriage takes place anyway.

Sometimes, age factors work in the opposite direction. Omar, a 73-year-old retired doctor, was contemplating marriage (his first) to a 69-year-old widow. His bride-to-be's children were concerned about the advanced years of both partners, and feared they, the children, would have to take on added responsibilities. Only after Omar pointed out his financial security, and his ability to hire experienced helpers should the need arise, did the future children-in-law give their blessings to the marriage.

Education

Education may become an issue in the family's approval of a marriage.

Education may also become an issue in the family's approval. The potential parents-in-law may decide that the children should complete their education before they marry, and may even make this a requirement before the marriage can take place. When a child decides to marry before earning a degree, it may be an annoyance to both sets of parents. Some fathers in therapy have demanded to know what the potential spouse is going to do to support their child, particularly if the child is a daughter. And, in these days when spouses are creating equal partnerships, sometimes the question is not "How will the husband support the wife?" but "Are both spouses able to support themselves, and, hence, the relationship?"

Family values differ regarding education. High-achieving parents may wonder what the in-law is going to do to gain more education. Blue-collar parents often feel threatened by a college-educated child-in-law. Family members may feel inferior, or fear they will be judged critically by the new addition to the family. Siblings-in-law may judge themselves against the new family member's job or degree. Blue-collar parents may also feel that the more-educated in-law is going to take their child away from them. Or, the new in-law may feel inferior throughout the relationship. For example, Patrice, a veterinary aide, said she did not think it bothered her that her husband had a law degree and she had only an associate's degree. But when they attended business functions, Patrice felt the situation was way over her head. "His sisters all hold master's degrees, so you can guess who never wants to play Trivial Pursuit™ at their parties," says Patrice. "I always heard that the wife rises to the social level of her husband, but I don't think it's true."

A Classless Society?

Although socioeconomic factors can be related to the education issue, the harsh reality of the myth that America is a classless society is all too often felt by in-laws who do not quite measure up to the newcomer's social standing. A child may bring into the family a potential in-law who is of a higher or lower socioeconomic status. If lower, the child may expect his or her family to help the incoming person to become more educated and more upwardly mobile. The parents-in-law might view these spouses as *projects*. In other words, the child brings home a spouse for the family to re-parent. Gus, a 62-year-old security guard, thought he would get along well with his son-in-law's family, but after going to their home for dinner, he was discouraged. "Their house is enormous, they have servants, and the place just reeks of old money," he said. "I don't know how we can ever even attempt to reciprocate socially."

Problems can arise when in-laws belong to different social classes.

If the socioeconomic disparity is too great, common ground between the families is rarely found. But we all need to be aware that social reciprocation need not be strictly equivalent. If one's family specializes in Tex-Mex barbecues, the blue-blooded in-laws may well enjoy being included.

Find a common ground and move forward without feelings of inferiority. Be yourself, and invite your new in-laws to join you as you enjoy life's pleasures.

The Power of Belief

Issues of marital compatibility are related to cultural or religious values.

Major issues of marital compatibility are often related to differences in cultural or religious values. In the heat of romance, many couples might disregard the fact that much of the family heritage is based on religious celebrations and rituals, especially when offspring enter the picture, and issues such as christening, catechism, communion, confirmation, baptism, or bar mitzvah must be addressed. Many people deny that they are religious and may say their religion has meant nothing to them for many years. They may even feel surprised at the importance they have suddenly given to their potential in-law's religious beliefs. But when it comes to their children's marriages, many parents suddenly find that they would like them to marry a Catholic, a Muslim, a Jew, or a Mormon, depending on their own religious background. Although some may deem this bigoted, there are some valid reasons for desiring religious compatibility.

For example, Jean, a 35-year-old writer, was brought up in a religious family, and her parents counseled her that "like should marry like." She did not realize how important her faith was until her first child was born. "I was heartsick that my husband, who is an agnostic, was unwilling to have our daughter christened in my church," she said. "Now, I'm teaching all my children the importance of marrying someone with the same belief structures they hold. I hope it will make a difference in *their* marriage choices."

Regarding religion and faith, make no assumptions about your in-laws or your partner. First find out what is important to them. Get to the specific details. It is usually the customs and not the doctrine that cause hang-ups. Then decide what is important to you. From both sides of the issues, determine where and how compromises can be made.

Ethnic Heritage

Ethnic background can become a volatile issue when a child is bringing a potential spouse into the home. The child who mistakenly thinks that his or her parents are liberal and understanding may be quite surprised at the reaction his or her choice of spouse might bring.

Ethnic background can become a volatile issue.

Although interracial marriage has become more common, parents-in-law often find it quite difficult to adapt to the interracial couple. The Oscar-winning film *Guess Who's Coming to Dinner* opened society's eyes a few decades ago; however, the old racial stereotypes continue to set families ablaze with conflict.

Ted and Barbara, who have been married for 30 years, met at the hospital where she was a nursing student and he was a medical resident. When she told her parents she was dating a doctor, they were thrilled, but then they found out that Ted was African American. Barbara's mother withheld her approval for the marriage; a month later, the couple wed with only Ted's parents in attendance. Barbara's mother did not speak to the couple for two years, but after their first child was born, she started to warm up to Ted, and, after 30 years and five children, she said that Ted has been a good son-in-law. "I give Ted credit for putting up with a lot," says Barbara.

We could look at every marriage as a *mixed marriage* because it brings together two people who, to some degree, have different customs, habits, and personalities. I have found that no matter how mixed the marriage, the initial acceptance of the bride into her husband's family (and vice versa) is a primary factor in how successful the marriage will be.

We could look at every marriage as a mixed marriage.

Quasi In-Laws—Those Unofficial Yet Integral Members of the Extended Family

Are they, or are they not your in-laws? If you have a grandchild or child who lives with a significant other, or who is in a serious relationship, you have in-laws, but since they are not in-laws by law, I describe them as *quasi* or *unofficial* in-laws.

I was recently interviewed by a young woman regarding my first book, *In-laws: A Guide to Extended Family Therapy*. She made a comment that she was not married and did not have in-laws. However, she lived with her boyfriend and had a very close relationship with his parents. She said it is difficult to be in the position of being in the family while not really feeling part of the family. She said she was not ready to call her unofficial in-laws *Mom* and *Dad*, as that presupposed more than she was ready for at that point in the relationship. I think *unofficial in-laws* is probably a good term to describe her relationship with her boyfriend's family.

However, if this woman and her partner had children, it would be a different matter. In the past, in some states after seven years, cohabitants were considered to be in a common-law marriage. This is no longer the case where no children are involved. You might want to check your state's laws to see what happens when you have children, and how the law then sees your relationship. When children are born, a friendship relationship with an unofficial in-law has an added biological bond. This would put it in a category entirely different from a strictly live-in relationship.

Many parents-in-law have different moral values than their children. Although there may be an unofficial in-law status, the parents-in-law may feel uncomfortable when children live together before marriage. They may not wish to acknowledge unofficial in-laws if they disapprove of the living arrangements. These issues need to be worked out on an individual basis and may need the help of a professional counselor.

Permission Granted: Welcome to the Clan

Do you desire to be a part of the family?

For you to be accepted by your in-laws, you must first have the desire to be a part of the family. Only then will the family gatekeepers, usually the parents-in-law, give you formal or informal permission to join the clan.

If you as a potential new in-law feel that there is resistance or that permission has not been given, you and your partner need to confront this directly, either on your own or with professional help. Only with permission, blessings, and welcome can the in-laws really move on to the acceptance and shared commonality that can bring family members closer.

You can understand why there are sayings such as, "You can choose your friends, but you can't choose your family." This is certainly true of in-laws. You can choose whom you will marry, but your in-law relationship is catch-as-catch-can. In many ways, in-laws are similar to associates at the office. You can choose to work for a firm, maybe even for a particular boss, but you cannot choose the majority of your co-workers. Your work situation may give you a clue about dealing with your in-laws. How do you interact in relationships that are not of your choosing? How do you get along with your fellow workers? What type of workers do you get along with? How do you best get along with them? If you have a lot of trouble with your fellow workers, you might compare that situation with your in-law problems. Ask yourself:

In-laws are similar to associates at the office.

- "What kind of environment or situation do I like to be in?"

- "Am I a loner and is that a problem?"

- "Am I on a computer at work all day and do I prefer not to interact with people?"

Look at yourself to identify what you bring to the in-law environment and the in-law space. If you are having work *and* in-law problems, are these problems more about you or those with whom you interact?

Consulting Others

Making decisions jointly with others in the family is an established method of getting along well with family members. When the relatives who are concerned are consulted, each feels in on the decision and shares responsibility for it. When the channels of communication are kept open between in-laws, real feelings can find expression, and hidden meanings are less common.

People who accept the fact that they do differ learn to resolve their conflicts in ways that protect—and respect—the values of each individual. Open discussion and mutual respect are recommended; however, with some in-laws, these goals may be too ambitious. A sincere willingness to see all possibilities and to avoid thinking there can be only one solution is important for your success at getting along with in-laws.

Where Do You Think You Are Taking My Daughter?

In therapy, I see two types of situations that arise when daughters start to date seriously or plan to be married. Some fathers come in and say, "I don't want my little girl to marry. We've always been close. I'm really going to miss her," or "I don't want her to steadily date a boy. I've always enjoyed having her as my little girl."

Preparation for letting a daughter move into a marriage and an adult female role starts during the girl's adolescence, when the father gives permission for his daughter to attend male–female activities and, later, to date. This transition into adulthood is hard for some daughters and fathers to negotiate, and can sometimes be hard for daughters and mothers, too.

I remember one father in therapy whose daughter was a high school basketball player. He enjoyed going to all of her games, coaching her, and being involved with her basketball team. When she decided in her senior year to drop off the team to spend more time with her studies and social activities, he was furious at her, and, indeed, even stopped speaking to her.

The daughter became extremely angry with him and started staying out late, drinking, and becoming generally rebellious. The family ended up coming into therapy, and we discussed the fact that she would be growing up, getting married, and moving into a new relationship that would place her father in the role of a father-in-law. The father began to see how he was living through his daughter and how he needed to develop a new relationship with her in order to enjoy his future son-in-law and grandchildren.

In therapy, I also see situations in which daughters begin to date or get serious about a young man, and mothers become controlling and restrictive of their daughter's moving into a new role that involves male companionship and possible future sons-in-law. Some women can be fairly provocative and jealous if they did not experience the kinds of relationships that their daughters are having with their boyfriends. With open communication, families can move toward better understanding of this transitional time.

Disclosure of Past Romantic Associations

Unfortunately, many marriages begin with problems relating to prior liaisons and breaches of conduct. Some newlyweds feel threatened by the discovery of one or more former romantic associations. This problem can be especially difficult if in-laws, friends, and family are aware of these earlier relationships. Prior to marriage, you might consider a frank dialogue with your partner in which you completely disclose to each other all former romantic associations. Each of you should give positive assurance that those relationships are completely ended, and agree that, thereafter, the former romantic relationships should never be brought up by either of you or by your families. Generally, such a discussion takes place privately between the couple; however, in some instances, the families may be involved or a therapist may be sought to help one or the other partner work through the intense feelings such disclosures engender. Being honest can have its risks, and each couple must decide what to do on an individual basis. However, if the in-laws are aware of past relationships, these secrets, if disclosed, can be destructive.

Consider disclosing all former romantic associations.

Common Knowledge

In some communities, there are "secrets" that the whole town knows. I grew up in a small town. My best friend Cleo lived on a farm outside of town. In the summer when we were 15 years old, she fell deeply in love with her father's hired hand. He was 21 and had drifted in to work for the family during the big harvesting season. Her parents were opposed to the relationship because of her age and because they saw him as only a drifter who was not part of our community.

One night, Cleo ran off with the farm hand to a state that required no waiting period, and they got married. It took her parents a couple of weeks to find Cleo. When they did, they told her in no uncertain terms that she could not stay in this marriage with the farm hand. They told the young man that if he persisted in this union, they would take him to court for statutory rape. The parents then initiated an annulment. The farm hand left, and Cleo never saw him again.

Cleo graduated from our local high school and went on to the university, where she met a young man, Derek. Cleo told Derek about her two-week marriage to the farm hand when she was 15. Derek was very understanding and supportive of Cleo. However, he chose not to tell his parents about Cleo's background. The couple got engaged and made their marital plans.

Several weeks prior to the marriage, a cousin of Cleo informed Derek's parents about Cleo's elopement with the farm hand. Derek's parents were outraged and felt that their son was getting someone who had not only been married but also was involved in a horrendous scandal. Cleo and Derek eventually married, but it took several years for the in-laws to accept the relationship and for the gossip to die down in the neighboring community. Fortunately, Cleo had told Derek about the relationship, and he was prepared to stand by her through his parents' disapproval.

This couple avoided the stress that can be placed on a marriage when one of the partners discovers that the other partner has had a theretofore undisclosed significant romantic association with someone who is, or might still be, involved in the couple's life.

Being with Family

Some people really enjoy being a part of an extended family. One young bride said that, although her husband did not like to spend time with extended family, she really enjoyed it. It was difficult for her to spend time with her own extended family because her husband would make comments to her like, "You're always running off to your parents," or "You're choosing between me and your family." But when she went to her in-laws' house, he was unable to say that she was choosing his family over him; instead, she was just being a part of the whole family situation. Even though he did not spend a lot of time with the family when he went there, she was able to enjoy her mother-in-law and siblings-in-law. It was important for this young woman to live near her in-laws, rather than her biological parents, because her husband made being with her own family an impossible situation.

As this marriage matures and the young woman feels more secure in her role, she may be able to divide her time more equally between her in-laws and her own family. She may communicate to her husband that a marital relationship is totally different from a parent–child relationship and loving in one does not mean taking love away from the other.

What Will We Call Each Other?

Have you experienced a problem with how to address your in-laws? When I married in the 1960s, I did not know what to call my in-laws. When we had a baby, I could at least call them Grandpa and Grandma. In American society at large, there is no change in name to designate a child's revised relationship to his or her parents after the child has married.

What should you call your in-laws?

However, in the Jewish and the Tongan cultures, there are name changes. Lack of a universal name may be due to the fact that this changed relationship has not been acknowledged as one of the significant forces in people's lives.

Jason asked his future father-in-law for his daughter's hand. His father-in-law gave him the third degree and wanted to know what he had done to deserve his *little girl*. After the wedding, Jason called his father-in-law "Sir" for the first year, until the parent took Jason aside and said, "The name is Bill." Jason said, "I really thought I had arrived."

Jason's distancing illustrates the quandary over what one should call a new in-law. If you think I am making a mountain out of a molehill, think again. These seemingly minor issues are often ignored but have been known to cause some major difficulties and tension.

Are they called Melvin and Tillie? Mom and Dad? Or Mr. and Mrs. Jenkins? The question of *What do we call you?* is usually not a problem for the parents-in-law (it is customary for them to call the daughter- or son-in-law by the first name), but many new children-in-law find it very difficult to approach the subject.

In a playful moment, I formulated the following name alternatives for the father-in-law, mother-in-law, and child-in-law, by dropping the "in-law" and the first letter of the title: *ather* for father, *other* for mother, and *hild* for child. Using new names would reinforce the change of status on a daily basis. More importantly, the new names would indicate symbolically a new dynamic in the relationship—something that does not happen following a one-hour ceremony. For those who find *other* offensive as a name for mother, consider these alternatives: *ad* for dad, *om* for mom, and *id* for kid! My options are playful but it is vital that, in the early stages, both the future parents-in-law and children-in-law address the situation with a long-term view and, when possible, accommodate the desires of others. A little warmth here will go a long way toward a loving relationship.

Planning the Wedding and the Ceremony

The day finally comes when a couple decides to marry. Ideally, by this point, the future in-law relationship is being successfully negotiated, because chances are high that the engagement and wedding planning stage will move even the most stable families toward chaos. Weddings are the source of myriad in-law problems and misunderstandings. Miss Manners, Elizabeth Post, and Amy Vanderbilt have tried to deal with these problems by issuing strict edicts of protocol. One of the best reasons for following these rules is that they can circumvent many problems with future in-laws.

Tensions run high at the time of weddings. Many decisions must be made and numerous factors need to be considered, such as flowers, cakes, dresses, location, type of wedding, and size of the guest list. The wedding is often a major social and financial event for the family, especially the bride's parents. Weddings seem to dredge up endless in-law jokes, such as: "What is the mother-in-law's place in the wedding? To wear beige and keep her mouth shut." Jokes like these can be painful for a woman who has been close to and involved with her child, especially if the bride or groom is an only child. Because responsibility for the planning of the wedding is closely connected to financial issues, those who foot the bill often have the ultimate say.

Tensions run high at the time of a family wedding.

Whose Wedding Is It, Anyway?

According to most etiquette guidelines, the wedding is the bride's; hence, the family of the bride is responsible for arrangements. However, if the family of the bride is not paying for the entire wedding, they often lose control of the event. In any case, there can be many hard feelings, slighted people, overlooked protocols, and missed deadlines. Petty annoyances can turn into major problems, particularly if the families are not mutually pleased with the choice of spouse.

Despite what many professionals in the wedding industry recite as absolute requirements for a correct and well-managed marriage ceremony and reception, the bride-to-be and the groom-to-be should have the ultimate responsibility for deciding what type of wedding celebration they are going to have. Accordingly, they should reach an agreement as to exactly how the marriage is to be celebrated, what range of cost is acceptable, and precisely who is to pay for each of the expenses incurred. Problems arise when assumptions are based solely on the practices of those who make their living in the wedding industry. Their concerns are centered on how many weddings they have booked for each season and how much they can enhance their profits through "must-have" extras. The desires and needs of the bride and groom and their parents are secondary to these salespeople. It is far wiser for the bride and groom to decide what type of ceremony and party they wish to have, and to reach a clear agreement regarding the budget and the schedule for payment. Couples who wait until the expenses have been incurred to make these decisions risk a disastrous relationship with the bride's parents or heavy overcharges on their own credit cards.

The same considerations hold true for the honeymoon. Many newlyweds find that, because of misunderstandings, their expectations regarding payment for the wedding, reception, and honeymoon have not been met. As a result, stress that could have been avoided is added to the new marriage. The bride-to-be and groom-to-be might find it wise to make a written agreement that itemizes the expenses of the wedding, reception, and honeymoon. If part of the expenses are to be borne by others (in most cases, this means the parents-in-law), the couple should have their agreement as well.

Who attends the wedding? Some of the early displays of disagreement may revolve around who attends the wedding. Guest lists can become a real bone of contention. The wishes of six people—the bride, the groom, and each of their parents (future in-laws)—must be considered regarding who should be invited. An additional decision is whether everyone on the guest list should be invited to both the wedding and the reception, or to just one.

Again, protocol can help: If it is agreed that etiquette makes it the bride's wedding, hard feelings can be avoided if the bride's wishes are considered first. However, the couple may want to start the relationship off on a happy note by honoring their future in-laws' requests.

Julie and Phil, two professionals who had been living together for two years, decided they would pay for their own wedding, with each of them taking equal responsibility. When Julie and her mother started to plan the wedding, a problem developed. Phil felt that he, rather than Julie's mother, should be involved in making the arrangements with Julie because his financial contribution allowed him to have equal input. During a therapy session with the couple, it became clear that Phil was seeking control but wanted to delegate all the work of the wedding to the two women. Julie pointed out that with decision making goes responsibility. Phil quickly decided to take a lesser role.

Dealing with Anger

Even with all family members trying their best, there will be slip-ups and major misunderstandings. I recently received a call from a woman I had seen in family therapy five years earlier. She asked if she and her husband could come in for a cooling-off session connected with her son's impending wedding. I said I would be delighted to see them again. As I hung up the telephone, I thought that her use of the word *impending* had an ominous quality.

It turned out that Mr. and Mrs. Reed had become especially angry when their son, Tom, showed them the wedding invitation. Having decided on a formal invitation, Meg, the bride, and her father had not included the groom's parents' names on the invitation. Because Tom was their first son, the Reeds felt slighted and upset. During the session, we discussed life cycle issues and I introduced the forming, storming, norming paradigm to the Reeds. (See Chapter 3.) The Reeds could definitely identify the wedding invitation as a storming stage issue and could see that their reaction (even though it might indeed have been justified) was putting undue pressure on Tom and placing them in an adversarial position with Meg. Mr. Reed admitted to some pride in wanting the fact that he was a professor to be reflected on the invitation. He also felt a lack of control regarding his son. He expressed loyalty to his wife's parents, saying that they had done a far better job of dealing with him 33 years earlier, at his own wedding. By the end of the session, Mr. Reed had calmed down considerably and left the session with the comment, "This too shall pass."

A week later, I got a call from Mrs. Reed. She said she wanted to let me in on something humorous. Apparently, when the couple had arrived home after the session, Mr. Reed pulled out their 33-year-old wedding book to show Tom how an invitation should look, and, to his surprise, found that his parents' names were not part of the invitation's wording. Mrs. Reed said they had enjoyed a good laugh with Tom, and a potential in-law misunderstanding was avoided.

Helping Families Sort It Out before They Become In-Laws—Overview

Our families are getting bigger, older, and more complicated. People are living longer and are healthier and more active than they were in the past. With today's high divorce and remarriage rates, blended families are increasing the spectrum of in-law relationships. How can parents-in-law and children-in-law see each other as resources and enhancements, rather than as annoyances and nuisances—or, in a more negative light, as destructive forces?

How do you go about sorting out the many dimensions of in-law relationship expectations? You can become intimidated by the whole prospect before a formal in-law relationship is even contemplated. Consider the following questions regarding your in-law relationships. Think of these questions in terms of yourself and then in regard to your family.

Worksheet

1. What are your perceptions and expectations about in-laws?

2. Do you like the way your father-in-law treats your mother-in-law (and vice versa)?

3. Have you recognized that you are marrying not just your spouse but his or her entire family?

4. What types of in-law relationships did you have in your biological family?

5. What changes in the family would the addition of an in-law make?

6. Do your parents-in-law (or your children-in-law) consider premarital sexual activity or cohabitation an issue?

7. Is giving in-laws permission (both verbal and nonverbal) to marry an issue in your family?

8. Have your future in-laws taken on the role of rejection?

9. Have you explored what it will mean in the long run if you or your family members do not accept the in-laws?

10. If you are getting married, is it clear who will take what roles in planning the wedding?

11. Have family members agreed on what the new parents-in-law will be called?

12. Have expectations regarding future or existing children been addressed, including the roles of in-laws and prior in-laws?

13. Are there unresolved issues around past romantic associations?

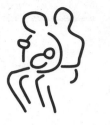

5

When Babies Enter the In-Law Picture

Big changes take place when children-in-law become parents.

Big changes take place in families when children-in-law become parents, parents-in-law become grandparents, and siblings-in-law become aunts and uncles.

Babies may give mothers-in-law, fathers-in-law, and siblings-in-law these new titles, but the advent of children into the extended family rarely clarifies the role played by these in-laws. Definitions of what it means to be a good parent-in-law or sibling-in-law are many and varied, and some relatives bring more sensitivity and common sense to the situation than others. New parents' feelings about the role of the new grandparents and other in-laws can range from a fear that they will be bad for the baby to a warm appreciation for the rich contribution they can make to their infant's life.

The new arrival can also put a strain on the relationship between the in-laws. The daughter-in-law can be put on the defensive very easily when her husband's mother or sister intrudes on her territory or shows her "how these things are done."

With longer life expectancies, grandparents are more numerous than ever before; about three-fourths of older people in the United States have living grandchildren. Of this number, nearly half see a grandchild almost every day. This grandparent contact indicates a high rate of in-law interactions. To my knowledge, no studies have reported on the quality of the in-law contact for grandparents, although grandparenting activities and expectations are often a source of in-law problems.

At the time of the birth of a first child, a couple's unresolved conflicts with their parents will often mushroom. The birth of a grandchild in some families is a signal for more active involvement of the in-laws and other extended family members in the young family's life, whether invited or not. Most aging men and women find it fairly easy to be the ideal grandparent when they see their grandchildren only occasionally. But when three generations live under the same roof, the charm of the youngest for the oldest is liable to wear off very soon—often, within days.

The Decision to Have a Child

Before the arrival of children, most married couples have reached an understanding regarding intentions and expectations of having children. It is easy to assume that a future spouse intends to participate in the birthing and rearing of children. Unfortunately, this assumption is often false. It is best for couples to have a clear agreement, prior to marriage, regarding child-rearing responsibilities. Parents-in-law can skew the equation with their expectations of becoming grandparents. Some in-laws actually compete for the status of being the first in the family to have a grandchild.

It is best for couples to have agreement, prior to marriage, regarding child-rearing responsibilities.

Barbara and Gary were engaged. Barbara was the youngest in a family of seven children and had long vowed that she would never have any children. Gary, an only child, had always dreamed of raising his own large brood, and he was deeply aware of his mother's regret that she could not have more babies. To further complicate things, Gary's mother and father were opposed to the marriage, because Barbara's firm no-child stance contradicted their strong desire for grandchildren. The couple sought therapy to help them come to an agreement they could both be happy with. I encouraged them to discuss their dreams and the pros and cons of having children. Gary admitted that, as an only child, he had always felt lonely. Barbara had the opposite problem with six older siblings. She had felt surrounded all her life and, because she had invested so much time and preparation, she did not want to sidetrack her career on the *mommy track*. The couple discussed ways that Gary could feel part of Barbara's large extended family. Gary acknowledged that he was not comfortable in close relationships with children. He decided to try to be the best brother-in-law and uncle possible, and the couple agreed to invite his mother and father to joint family activities attended by Barbara's siblings. Barbara said she would consider the possibility of having children in the future but, as she put it, only on a one-at-a-time basis. Gary also decided to tell his parents to back off on the grandparenting comments. Seven years later, when Barbara felt secure in her career, the couple decided to have a child, and Gary admits that the reality of caring for just one child has significantly altered his dreams of a large family.

Impatient In-Laws

Parents-in-law may be involved not only in the care and nurturing of grandchildren, but also in the actual timing of a grandchild's birth. One young couple, Lizabelle and Garth, came to my office especially frustrated because Garth's mother had clearly stated that she felt her son should quit school and that her daughter-in-law, Lizabelle (age 26), should get pregnant right away while the biological clock was still ticking. Garth's parents were divorced. Garth's father, who was paying his son's tuition, felt that his daughter-in-law should not get pregnant until his son had graduated from college. The two conflicting messages from his parents confused the son and infuriated his wife, who was from France and desired to re-create her own family within the United States. The couple's solution was to stop using birth control and to "let nature take its course." I last spoke to Lizabelle several months ago. She was not yet pregnant.

Currently, many couples are either dating longer or living together, creating a period of time when there may be an informal in-law relationship without children. In-laws in these circumstances can get fairly impatient and may wonder aloud when the couple will decide to get married or to have a child. The birth of a child greatly changes the family dynamics, because the child is an affirmation of life together and an addition to the family's history. Parents-in-law (and siblings-in-law, although to a lesser extent) can be very impatient about having the opportunity to move into the grandparenting role.

Naming the Baby—When In-Laws Get Involved

With a new baby expected in the family, in-law loyalty issues begin to surround the question: "What shall we name the baby?" Sharon and Cliff came to therapy for help in settling a family dispute. After learning through amniocentesis that their expected child would be a boy, they announced this to the parents-in-law. Sharon was incensed when her father-in-law emphatically demanded, "Of course, you will name him Clifford Blake Rutherford IV." Sharon's husband, who as the "III" and was tired of being referred to as "Little Cliff," was adamantly opposed. The conflict diminished the new parents' excitement and joy about an event that would not even take place for another five months. Sharon also feared that her father-in-law's stance signified future meddling and efforts to control.

What shall we name the baby?

I convinced the entire family to attend a therapy session, and we discussed what children mean in the family life cycle and the changes the birth would bring. A chart of the family history drew out reminiscence of an earlier power struggle between the father-in-law and his own father, which was being mirrored in his demands regarding his expected grandson. The mother-in-law interjected here that she had been reluctant to bestow on her son a III appellation, but had been conned into submission by her father-in-law and had resented it ever since. The family decided that the time had come to break with tradition. This allowed Sharon to graciously offer to give the baby the father-in-law's first name as his middle name.

The family was gratified that they had made the effort to resolve this issue, because the baby was born with major birth defects and died shortly after birth. When I called to offer my condolences, Sharon reflected with bittersweet irony that the conflict over the name actually brought her closer than ever to her parents-in-law and this bond was helping enormously in the grieving process.

In-Laws as Grandparents, Aunts, and Uncles

Before the grandchild is born, in-law relationships may revert to a storming stage.

Even before the grandchild is born, in-law relationships may revert to a storming stage, starting with such issues as illness, morning sickness, miscarriages, and the possibility of increased need of resources such as money and help with babysitting.

Rubin and Rhonda, a couple I saw in therapy, were extremely angry with their extended family. Rhonda had been bedridden for much of her pregnancy and was upset that she did not receive more attention from her mother-in-law. A rift developed between Rubin and his parents when he carried the message from his wife that his parents were not helpful or sympathetic enough. When the baby was six months old, Rhonda felt the need to punish the in-laws by not letting them see the child on a regular basis. During therapy, Rhonda was able to express her anger and hurt, but then realized that withholding access to the child was counterproductive. As Rubin pointed out to Rhonda, "The least they can do to make it up is to give us some free babysitting." Rhonda laughed and said she would ease up. When I last spoke to them, the couple said the situation was better and the baby loved his grandparents.

Perceptions of Being a Grandparent, Aunt, or Uncle

Most of us have not thought much about what kind of a grandparent, aunt, or uncle we want to be, or whether we had a choice. We just wait until the event happens. Our own personality and attitude, or the styles of our own grandparents, aunts, and uncles, are perpetuated almost unconsciously. But it is possible to make a conscious choice about what kind of a valued elder relative we can and want to be. For brevity, I have framed the discussion in terms of the grandparent role; however, the issues apply equally to aunts and uncles.

Misunderstandings can arise when parents-in-law behave toward their grandchildren in a way that children-in-law found objectionable in their own grandparents. A wise family discusses expectations of what a grandparent is or is not.

What kind of grandparent do you want to be? What kind of grandparents do you expect your in-laws to be? If the baby has already arrived, are you happy with your role as grandparent? Are you happy with your in-laws' roles as grandparents? To help assess what can happen when in-laws become grandparents, we can look at Helen Kivnick's book, *The Meaning of Grandparenthood.* Kivnick found that people's thoughts about being grandparents fit into five categories. I have added a sixth: reluctant grandparent. The categories are:

What kind of grandparents do you expect your in-laws to be?

1. **Centrality:** For these individuals, grandparenthood activities and feelings become more important as other activities and close friends and relatives become less important.

2. **Valued elder:** The focus for these grandparents is on passing their skills and traditions on to their grandchildren, and having the grandchildren think kindly of them and regard them as wise.

3. **Immortality through the clan:** These individuals see grandparenthood in terms of personal immortality, achieved through the continuity of their families into the indefinite future.

4. **Reinvolvement with personal past:** Being a grandparent lets these people remember when they were grandchildren, or when they were parents with children the same ages as their grandchildren are today.

5. **Indulgence:** These grandparents treasure the opportunity to *spoil* their grandchildren and to be more lenient and less critical than they were with their own children. This is a familiar in-law-loyalty problem area.

6. **Reluctant grandparent:** These grandparents are not ready to make the transition from parent or in-law to grandparent.

Styles of In-Law Grandparenting

Styles of in-law grandparenting vary.

Besides thinking of yourself and your in-laws in terms of your personal perception of grandparenting roles, you might find objective descriptions of styles of in-law grandparenting useful. In a study of grandparents of teenage children, researchers Andrew Cherlin and Frank Furstenberg identified the following four styles of grandparenting:

1. **The detached grandparent:** A distant figure, often a paternal in-law, who is not involved with the grandchildren.

2. **The passive grandparent:** Inactive, but functions by just being around. This grandparent may be filling the role that Lillian Troll terms *the family watchdog*.

3. **The influential grandparent:** More often than not, a maternal in-law. Sees children often and is a major figure in the grandchildren's day-to-day lives.

4. **The selective investment grandparent:** Turns his or her attention to a selected grandchild in order to make up for a poor relationship with other grandchildren.

Which style describes you? Are you happy or comfortable in that style? Which other style might you want to explore as a grandparent? Be aware that these are not set in stone. You will not always be 100 percent detached. Consider how you might wish to change. For example, if you realize that you have become a *selective investment* grandparent through the fluke of geographic distance, or that you are paying more attention to one set of grandchildren than another, you may decide to write letters and send cards to those who are far away. Consider making a videotape of grandpa and grandma and asking the grandchildren to reciprocate.

Being Supportive

In-laws and parents often have more child-rearing experience than the new parents and must try hard not to be too critical of them or to offer too much unsolicited advice. Depending on geographic proximity, experience, and attachment to children, parents-in-law may be more or less involved with the discipline or nurturing of the grandchildren. A *too good* in-law grandparent criticizes the new parent for not taking good enough care of the child—not feeding it enough or feeding it too much, diapering too tightly, or not changing the baby often enough and inviting diaper rash. The issue of whether to let the baby cry or pick up the baby can cause long-term rifts between parents and grandparents or siblings-in-law. As an in-law, curb negative, casual comments where children are concerned. Try to be an adviser—not a decision maker.

As an in-law, try to curb negative, casual comments where children are concerned.

Us Against Them

Humorist Sam Levinson said, "The reason grandparents and grandchildren get along so well is that they have a common enemy."

In-laws may enjoy having the child as their ally against the *bad parent*, but, in the long run, the entire family suffers. Everyone enjoys being right, but it is sometimes more important to be supportive than to be right. In-laws who band together with grandchildren risk alienating the parents to a point where they may lose contact with the young family.

Be sensitive to the parent–child relationship.

Enlightened in-laws should be sensitive to the parent–child relationship and should consult with the parents before making suggestions or making plans directly with their grandchildren, nieces, or nephews. By making the mother and father active participants in planning, the threats of envy and jealously are largely avoided.

Critical In-Laws

Some siblings-in-law and parents-in-law are highly critical of their sibling's or children's parenting skills and are in competition with the parents. In-laws may not be willing to childproof their house by removing breakables, and may get upset when shoes are on the furniture or fingerprints are on the walls. When such incidents occur, these critical in-laws blame the parents for failing to train their children correctly. If you are one of these critical in-laws, your grandchildren are probably rare visitors.

On the other hand, there *are* some inconsiderate children-in-law who let their youngsters get out of control and who allow them to destroy valuable possessions or to eat in nondesignated areas. Deal with these issues carefully and with tact. Seemingly insignificant comments can have long-lasting consequences.

Disciplining Your In-Law's Children

A number of issues surround discipline.

A number of issues surround discipline and general attitudes on the best ways to care for children. As a new aunt, Kelly, a 29-year-old teacher, was annoyed with how her sister-in-law was treating her son. "She spanks his hand constantly and tells him he's bad," said Kelly, "but my nephew is only three years old and I'm a third-grade teacher and I understand developmental issues." Kelly told her that time-outs were a better way to deal with this behavior, but the sister-in-law refused to listen.

Discipline of other people's children can be a challenge. One woman's granddaughter, Rachael, who was three years old, could sometimes get rather rowdy, and pulled the grandmother's hair or gave her a little punch in the face. When this happened, the grandmother gave Rachael a time-out and, fortunately, that response was all right with her daughter-in-law and son. Prior to babysitting, my client asked her daughter-in-law and son if they would mind if she disciplined Rachael in gentle ways. Having been given that permission, she enjoyed the relationship, and Rachael, knowing that there were boundaries with her grandmother, behaved accordingly.

Grandparenting as a Hobby, Not a Career

In-laws sometimes need to be reminded that the role of grandparenthood is not a career, but can be a delightful hobby when the parents are able to assume the role of primary caregivers. For some parents-in-law, grandparenting becomes a career because, through the parents' default, they become surrogate parents.

Grandparenthood is not a career.

Evelyn R. Duvall found that the grandparents in her study usually got themselves into emotional hot water with the family for the following reasons: (1) they did not keep up-to-date; (2) they interfered in the disciplining of the children, and (3) they became a threat to the mother when she perceived that her children loved the grandparents too much. I believe that the complaint of loving the grandparents too much stems from the child's getting more love and attention than the mother or dad got from these same people a generation ago.

In one young family, the paternal grandmother had become ill and moved in with her son and daughter-in-law and their two daughters,

Jesse (10) and Kristy (14). Jesse loved the grandmother very much and felt very close to her. Kristy, a typical adolescent, resented the grandmother's intrusion and felt that sharing the house with the grandmother was a real imposition on the family. She constantly bad-mouthed her grandmother, and tension and friction were created in the home. Kristy may have mirrored some of the attitudes of the mother, who was not happy about having her mother-in-law in the home. No doubt, Kristy was being allowed to express her anger because it reflected the anger of her mother. During the course of therapy, it became evident that the mother-in-law was seen as an intrusion in the home. I encouraged the husband to understand the conflict that revolved around his mother's presence. I also sought to bring in his three other siblings. The family agreed that it was not fair for this one family unit to bear the entire burden of the mother-in-law. It was arranged that she would rotate among her four children, moving from one home to the next on a quarterly basis. This is not an ideal situation for an older, ill person. However, the mother-in-law was willing to cooperate in order to maintain the goodwill of her granddaughter and daughter-in-law.

Grandparents as a Resource

Children need grandparents to add richness, perspective, and fullness to life. Grandparents serve a real purpose in providing for children a different relationship than the parent–child bond. Often, grandparents can take time to listen and, because they are usually not responsible for the child on a day-to-day basis, can afford to be less judgmental.

Grandparents can enjoy their grandchildren with unique freedom. When they brought up their own children, they were bound by the expectations and demands of parenthood. They are free to enjoy their grandchildren as persons.

Ideally, children-in-law will be aware of the importance of grandparents in their children's lives, and parents-in-law will realize that grandparenting children is a privilege and not a right. When driving a car, someone who follows the rules and does not make too many mistakes is allowed on the highway. Grandparents who follow the rules set by the custodial caregiver (usually, the parent) will be allowed the privilege of grandparenting.

Protecting the Relationship with Grandchildren

Therapists often see a situation where grandparents do not feel they have enough access to their grandchildren. I saw one case that was particularly difficult. Robert told me that he was having problems with his parents-in-law. They had been rude to his wife and she reciprocated by not allowing them access to their grandchildren. Quite a rift had been created, and Robert asked if I would see them all. The father, mother, and daughter (Robert's wife) had a long history of problems and anger toward one another.

Access to grandchildren is not a given.

As the son-in-law, Robert felt that the children should not be punished because of this ongoing conflict. He was anxious for the grandchildren to have a good relationship with his in-laws. During the course of therapy, he was able to state this and to say that he was really tired of hearing about childhood problems. He felt that the children deserved to have a good relationship with their grandparents as well as with their parents, and he would love to start, here and now, to work on those relationships. Robert also said that he wanted his children to have a good role model for dealing with grandparents. He was afraid that the same kinds of things that were happening with the grandparents now would be repeated when he was a grandparent.

I suggested that his parents-in-law (the grandparents) take the role of experienced advisers, people who give advice only when asked and do not insist on it being taken. I reminded them of the mutual love they had for the young children, and they agreed to call a truce in their relationship and concentrate on parenting and grandparenting issues. When I last checked, they were still having problems on and off, but Robert said that things had greatly improved and that his wife was much more willing to let the grandparents be more involved with the children.

Religious Issues

Religious ceremonies can be an area of friction.

Grandchildren bring out some of our most basic caring and love, as well as our concern that things be done for them in a way that we deem appropriate. Religious ceremonies can be an area of friction if compromise cannot be reached. For example, Lydia's daughter-in-law was Catholic. Lydia, who was not Catholic, objected to the baby's being christened in a Catholic ceremony. She decided that, rather than fight the idea, she and her daughter-in-law might combine their two cultures by baptizing the baby in the Catholic Church and just giving it a name and a blessing in Lydia's church. Lydia proposed this to her son first and got his permission to approach her daughter-in-law with the idea.

Fortunately, Lydia's son and daughter-in-law agreed to having the baby involved in the rituals of two separate religions. This outcome is not usual. Coming up with innovative ideas can be risky, but rewarding.

Advice for New Parents

After several weeks of nonstop care of a new baby, husbands and wives really need to have some Couple's Time. To do this, they might ask for an in-law's help. Studies have shown that marital satisfaction decreases with the birth of children and increases again as the children become older. A grandparent's, or an aunt's or uncle's involvement can be very helpful when they can take the children for activities so the couple can have some intimate time together.

As a new parent, one way to really annoy siblings-in-law is to bring infants and young children to events where they are not welcome. There are adult events and there are events where children are included. Do not assume that your siblings-in-law want your children at their

Christmas party or at a wedding reception. Be courteous. Ask if an event is appropriate for the nephews and nieces, and if the answer is no, do not be offended. Do not sacrifice your relationship with your in-laws out of pride in your offspring. Remember, as nephews and nieces, your children will get to know and love your siblings-in-law soon enough.

Advice for New Grandparents

I asked Bonnie, a friend who has five children and twelve grandchildren, for her advice to a new grandmother. She said that grandparents need to be aware that it is impossible to treat all grandchildren equally. They must be careful what they do for and with the first grandchild because their kids and in-laws will keep score. "If you're going to put some money in the bank for every birthday, realize that as it comes down the line to 12 grandchildren, the expenses will really add up." She advises grandparents to avoid making promises or doing things for the first grandchild that they are not going to be able to do as other grandchildren join the clan. "It's such a thrill to have the first grandchild, and you want to do so many things . . . , but by the time you have 12 grandchildren and you've given $100 for each birthday, you're on the hook for $1,200 a year," said Bonnie. "If you don't follow through with each grandchild, it really drives a wedge between you, your children, and your in-laws."

Expectations of Child Care and Baby-Sitting

Elderly people who have not planned for their retirement and do not have much money sometimes end up baby-sitting for their children in order to pay their rent or in exchange for being able to live with their children. In the past, in-laws were *expected* to provide child care and baby-sitting. More families lived with several generations under the same roof, and the in-laws were natural baby-sitters because they were always available. I remember wonderful times in my childhood when I sat under

Child care and baby-sitting are no longer in-law activities.

the weeping willow trees with my grandmother and my great-grand-mother, drinking lemonade as though they had nothing else in the world to do but take care of me. It just seemed to be a foregone conclusion that grandmothers would do a great deal of baby-sitting.

Expecting in-laws to baby-sit today may be unrealistic. Our lifestyle is much more fast-paced. Many in-laws are working, traveling, or involved in other activities that take them out of the baby-sitting realm. Where families are no longer living together, the babysitter will not have the children's equipment, toys, books, and beds at his or her house. Your situation, the culture of your in-laws, and your own ideas about baby-sitting all feed into your decision on who stays with your children when you go out.

Ellen, a 37-year-old paralegal, was thankful for her in-laws' generosity. She explained that her parents-in-law did not have very much money to help the couple out when they got married, but one of the best gifts they ever gave was their offer to take care of the grandchildren while Ellen and her husband worked. Ellen said it was so comforting to know that her babies were being well cared for, and the family was able to save up enough money to buy a house just three years after the wedding. "I recently told my husband, 'Your folks' gift of time was more precious than gold,'" said Ellen.

Child care and baby-sitting can create many disagreements because of different expectations among in-laws. If the woman is the primary care-giver, she may have minimal conflict when her own parents take care of the children, because they may have similar caregiving standards and behaviors. However, if she resents the way her parents brought her up, she may resist having them mind her children.

If there are many problematical child-rearing issues, it might be good to go over in detail the grandparents' methods of discipline and their eating and bedtime schedules, particularly if the parents are leaving the children with the in-laws overnight. When I work with couples who are separating or are divorced and whose children go from one house to the other, I always suggest that they make one schedule and keep the children on it no matter where they are staying.

Expecting grandparents to adhere to a rigid schedule can create difficulty. Because their circumstances are different, the in-laws may want to take the children out and come home later, or they may let them sleep in. I recommend that parents be flexible when children are being cared for by grandparents. A lot of friction can surround issues as small as letting young children drink carbonated drinks or eat cookies. When children come home and report what their grandparents let them do, in-laws can get extremely upset if they feel those things are taboo. Baby-sitters must be informed regarding signs of medical emergencies or schedules for children's medication. One client told me she was furious that her mother-in-law had given her child cough syrup, because she did not want her child to have anything with alcohol.

When Babies Arrive on the In-Law Scene— Overview

New arrivals on the in-law scene provide plenty of opportunity for missed communications, stepped-on toes, and bad feelings, as well as an unlimited potential for joy, richness, and fun. How your in-law situation weathers the arrival of children depends on the perspectives and expectations of the players involved. Luckily, most children arrive ready to be loved and nurtured, and they are generally more than willing to be the recipients of affection from all interested parties. The new roles adopted can be either positive or negative. It helps when both children-in-law and parents-in-law have clear ideas of age hierarchies and the responsibilities that go with them.

Have clear ideas and responsibilities.

If you, as a parent, have primary responsibility for bringing a new child into the world and raising this tiny person into successful adulthood, you will soon recognize that nobody can do it alone. You will need plenty of help all along the way. If you are a sibling-in-law, the child's entrance gives you the opportunity to master the art of being an aunt or uncle. Will you be seen as wise, witty, wonderful, loving, and adventurous, or "that old crank who is always asking when she's going to get her thank-you note"?

And if you, as a parent-in-law, have already raised your children to adulthood, you now have the pleasure of welcoming a new grandchild into your family circle. How can you, as an in-law, gracefully negotiate this life cycle change? One of the most helpful ideas is that being with grand-children is a privilege, not a right. The corollary for new parents is: View the grandparents as a valuable resource that can meaningfully add to the life of your child, and avoid taking advantage of or abusing the in-laws' willingness to be with their grandchildren. Mutual respect goes a long way toward smoothing the in-law path when children arrive.

This chapter is intended to give readers a chance to assess perceptions of being a grandparent, aunt, or uncle, and to help in-laws develop a sound style and a plan. Being an in-law grandparent can be both rewarding and satisfying when peace reigns among the parents-in-law, children-in-law, and grandchildren.

The following list of questions will help identify potential trouble spots. Your answers can generate discussion and decisions about the changes that come about with the addition of children to the in-law spectrum. For all the questions, substitute "aunt" or "uncle" for grandparent, as appropriate for your situation.

Worksheet

1. How do your perceptions of a grandparent fit with your in-law's?

2. Is an in-law's attendance at the childbirth an option? If you would like to attend the delivery, have you discussed it with the parents, especially the mother?

3. Would you like to have or participate in home help from in-laws after the birth of the child? Have you discussed who will visit or set up an in-law visitation schedule after the baby has gone home?

4. As an in-law, how can you be supportive of first-time parents' parenting skills?

5. Do you as a grandparent try to remain neutral and avoid taking sides with children against their parents?

6. In what ways can you be sensitive to the fact that grandparenting is a privilege, not a right?

7. Do you try to be a resource to your children-in-law or siblings-in-law, and hold back on advice?

8. Are you avoiding parents-in-law and children-in-law competition?

9. Are you aware that the parents-in-law's infertility or decreased virility can cause friction between the generations?

10. Do you, as an in-law, expect to be involved in occasional baby-sitting or regular full-time day care of your grandchildren or nieces and nephews? Have you discussed expectations?

6

Changing Tides—Aging and the In-Law Relationship

In-Laws' Role Changes

Milestones like the natural aging process impact the in-law relationship.

Almost no attention has been devoted to in-law relationships in the later years of the life cycle. However, many seemingly typical events can disrupt and redefine the expectations of in-law relationships. Such milestones as the addition of children, divorce, illness, grandparent-hood, the natural aging process, the need to be cared for, death, and other expected and unexpected events will certainly impact the in-law relationship.

To be healthy and to survive, the in-law system must be flexible, allowing for change, growth, and the introduction of new roles. One young man in therapy told me that his parents and his wife's parents had taken care of them all their lives, and so, at 30 years of age, he felt it was time for him to be the man of the house and to start taking care of his parents and parents-in-law. I pointed out that caring is mutual and empowers all people involved in giving to others. At different ages, however, people have different needs and responses—advancing age does not mean that in-laws or parents desire or need to be *taken care of*. The opposite also applies: Just because one is 30 years of age does not mean that one cannot accept some caring from in-laws and/or parents. There are times when we can give support and times when we need support.

Parents' New Roles as Experienced Advisers

Early in my career as a therapist, I used to talk about parents-in-law as being *trusted advisers*. Then an in-law came in who had not been a particularly good father and had not been available for his daughter or his son-in-law but had depended on them for money and a place to stay. I decided that not all parents were trusted advisers, but they were *experienced advisers*. If nothing else, parents have been through the early life stages the young couple is experiencing.

As mentioned earlier, I now suggest that parents-in-law assume the role of experienced advisers, remembering always that advisers give advice only when asked or when called upon. Children-in-law who see their parents-in-law in the role of experienced advisers should also recognize the value of this role and give them the opportunity to be advisers by asking for some advice. Advisers must always remember that their advice will not necessarily be taken.

Parents-in-law assume the role of experienced advisers.

Many family life cycle issues are highly predictable, in terms of changes for the family and in-laws. In their groundbreaking book on the family life cycle, Elizabeth Carter and Monica McGoldrick have formulated a six-stage family life cycle.

When a couple moves through those six stages, these are the related in-law tasks:

Stages	In-Law Tasks
1. Fred is 28 and single, and seriously dating Sue.	Introducing sibling-in-law relationships into the family.
2. Fred makes a commitment to Sue. They are living together or married.	Possibly negotiating an experienced adviser role for parents and in-laws.
	(continued)

(Continued)
Stages   *In-Law Tasks*

3. Fred and Sue become parents.   Enlarging the in-law roles to include
                                                                      grandparenting and experienced adviser
                                                                      status.

4. Fred and Sue's children move into   Beginning to shift concerns toward older
   adolescence.   generation, including parents-in-law.
                                                                      Older generation and younger generation
                                                                      have the possibility for a special bonding.

5. The children leave home; this means   Renegotiating relationships to include
   an empty nest for Fred and Sue.   children's marriages, with a second
                                                                      generation of new in-laws, plus
                                                                      grandchildren and grandparenting roles.

6. Fred and Sue become senior citizens.   Sharing of wisdom and ideas by elderly
                                                                      in-laws. Children-in-law are supportive
                                                                      while not taking over for elderly in-laws,
                                                                      thus keeping them competent.

The In-Law Life Cycle—Awareness of Expected and Unexpected Life Events

It is sometimes difficult for parents-in-law to see when it is time to gear down, step aside, and, in a quiet way, let the younger generation take over some of the work. Especially for some fathers-in-law, who are used to an authoritarian role, problems can arise when there is a family business involved. A play I recently saw illustrates how authoritarian men have difficulty passing the mantle to the younger generation. *Hobson's Choice*, by Harold Brighouse, is about an elderly widowed shopkeeper with three daughters who marry during the course of the play. When left to live alone, Hobson, an alcoholic, begins to suffer ill health. The doctor recommends that Hobson have one of his daughters and her husband move in with him. The oldest daughter is the only one willing to make the move—out of *duty*. The son-in-law (her husband) had worked for Hobson as a bootmaker, and Hobson sees him as a mere functionary. In the end, the daughter and son-in-law move in, but only after Hobson agrees, under duress from the couple, to make his son-in-law an equal partner in the shop. The other two daughters are outraged that their portion of the shop will slip from their hands to their brother-in-law and sister; however, they are not willing to pay the price of taking care of the old man.

This play, set in the late 1800s, echoes an enduring in-law theme. For example, William, an 80-year-old retired restaurateur, was in business with his son-in-law, Dick. The restaurant had been in William's family for two generations, and Dick, who managed the concern, wanted to establish a franchise. William was against it, and it caused a rift between them. However, Dick established a very successful franchise operation. "I predicted a bankruptcy," said William. "It has been ten years now and I hate to admit that I was dead wrong." Although chagrined, William threw his support behind his son-in-law's efforts and they have since become a terrific example of the graceful passage of the reins in a business.

Retirement

People are living longer than at any time in our history; older Americans are no longer relegated to a rocking chair on the porch. With the increasing numbers of seniors, the activities and options concurrently expand.

Retirement is certainly not the end of life, and in this era of early retirement packages, reductions in workforce, and mandatory retirement, many people are retiring earlier than ever before. Along with the fact that they are healthy, many look forward to a second career. For in-laws, the necessary adjustment can be difficult. An in-law who had always

It takes a couple of years to adjust to retirement.

been working is now around all the time and is trying to adjust to retirement. That adjustment can take a couple of years. New interests may develop, or, after a taste of retirement, the retiree may seek a part-time job. Even if you do not live in the same area as the in-law, this life cycle change often impacts the children-in-law, because they may be called or visited by the in-laws more frequently.

It is never too late to start a career, and your in-laws may surprise you with their postretirement energy. On the other hand, you may be saying to yourself, "How do I get *my* in-laws to get this kind of energy and do the things that you are talking about?" They may not have any desire to get out and be active. They may prefer to sit and watch the soaps, or sleep, or eat or drink a lot. When people have made it through 50 or 60 years, I think one has to let them decide to live their lives at their own pace. You can make recommendations, but chances are they will do what they want to do.

Most people will treat you the way you let them know that you want to be treated.

During these times of change, identify how you would like to see yourself as an in-law, and how you would like others to see you, can be a highly empowering process. In my view, most people will treat you the way you let them know that you want to be treated. Let's face it: Most of us are basically lazy. We do not want to aggravate people or create problems. If people let us know their limits, or the way they want to be treated, we will often try to be compliant and treat them in that way.

Parents-in-law and children-in-law need to give some thought as to how they would like to be treated as they age.

We should all make a conscious effort to deal with problem areas in our lives. Keeping our elderly population empowered and working with them on being and feeling needed can greatly enhance our lives. They are a tremendous resource of knowledge as well as support. As parents-in-law live longer and enjoy better health, it is wise to capitalize on their strengths and encourage them to continue to be independent and functional. Many of my older clients express the thought that their extended family members have difficulty realizing that even though they may be *older* or *over the hill*, they still have hopes, dreams, desires, and (surprise!) plans for the future.

As you go through your own life cycle, you might want to ask, "Have I given myself and others the permission to grow and change through the family life cycle, or do we have to reach some kind of predicted age of retirement?"

Illness of an In-Law

Another life cycle problem that can stress the family is the illness of an in-law—most often, an aging parent-in-law. With the advent of nursing homes, some of this care of the elderly is now left to professionals. However, for some in-laws, taking care of an elderly or ill relative is a satisfying experience. Lori told me she was very close to Glenda, her mother-in-law, who at age 65 was diagnosed with stomach cancer. On the day she was told by the doctor, Lori told her, "Glenda, I will never put you into a nursing home. I will take care of you." This created a strong bond and closeness between the two. Lori had the support of her husband, who was very close to his mother. As a family, Lori and her husband took care of Glenda for two years, until she died at home in her bed. "We had some rough times taking care of her, but I will never regret the time that my husband and I had with her," said Lori. "She was a wonderful mother-in-law and a good friend." The care of an infirm elderly relative at home is the exception rather than the rule. Many families are not able to care for elderly in-laws.

Illness of an aging parent-in-law can stress the family system.

When Is It Time for a Nursing Home or Hospice Program for In-Laws?

What to do with an ill or incapacitated in-law is always a difficult dilemma. Finances and insurance can greatly impact an in-law's decisions.

In addition to a range of age-related health problems, Alzheimer's disease makes a serious impact on the care of elderly in-laws. Nancy Mace and Peter Rubins, in *The 36-Hour Day*, explore at-home care of people who have Alzheimer's disease, and give some excellent suggestions on how to deal with in-laws. Another resource is *Alzheimer's Disease: A Guide for Families* by Lenore S. Powell, which describes what to expect as Alzheimer's progresses.

Most people would like to stay at home and never enter a nursing home or a hospice program, but this is not always possible. My experience shows that most people are able to keep their incapacitated family members at home until they do not sleep through the night. Home care then becomes extremely difficult. With strokes, dementia, or Alzheimer's disease, some affected in-laws become combative and at times hostile. My own parents lived in a condominium. One night, my father opened the bedroom window and started screaming out, "Help, help, she's killing me." At that point, my mother sadly decided that she had to put him in a nursing home. This was not something she wanted to do. However, when she went to visit the nursing home, she realized that many of the people they had known growing up in their small town were now residing in the nursing home and that thought offered some amount of comfort.

A good nursing home is not a place that warehouses; it is a place that works with people to keep up their emotional, physical, and intellectual capacities. *Consumer Reports* published an excellent series of articles in 1995 on how to choose a nursing home. Reprints are available by writing CU/Reprints, 101 Truman Avenue, Yonkers, NY 10703-1057.

A lot of guilt is connected with putting an in-law or a spouse in a nursing home. To ease their guilt, some children-in-law will resort to telling their family member that he or she will be going home soon, although in reality the home has been sold and the contents have already been sold or divided. I encourage family members to tell the truth about the circumstances. Not telling people the truth can cause much unhappiness.

The Empty Nest Fills—Children-in-Law Living with Parents-in-Law

In this age of expensive housing, prolonged education, and changes in circumstances, it is not unusual to see young couples coming and going from their parents' family home. Just when parents-in-law thought they were home free and their children were launched, they may find themselves with a house full of adult children and their in-laws (and sometimes their grandchildren).

Move In and Pitch In

It is one thing to be a guest and stay with a friend for two or three days. It is quite another to move in with your in-laws. The in-laws who move in must remember that the need for scrubbing floors, cleaning bathrooms, and washing towels is greatly increased by having more people living in the home; as residents, they should feel responsible for a share of the work. It may seem magical to arrive home from work and find the house clean, but someone's efforts have made it that way. Try surprising your in-laws by occasionally helping out financially: buy some groceries or pay some utility bills. Be prepared to reimburse your hosts for any long-distance telephone charges you incur. Or, if the in-laws do not want financial help, do the minimum: keep your own belongings neat and tidy and your own area clean. Cleaning a bathroom, picking up towels, changing light bulbs, and running a vacuum cleaner can all be very helpful activities, so pitch in if you want the welcome mat to stay out.

An In-Law's Death

The death of a family member can create havoc in the family, especially if there is a family estate or family home to be disposed of. In-laws can get overly curious and sometimes inappropriately involved in times of crisis. Untimely deaths, such as the death of a child, represent enormous trauma for families, and everyone wants to rush in and help. Tensions run high when a funeral must be planned and visitors must be housed. Hurtful things said by in-laws and other family members at these times are not soon forgotten.

Death or illness of a family member tests the strength and flexibility of an extended family.

Death or illness of a family member tests the strength and flexibility of an extended family and can be highly disruptive to in-law relationships. Sarah felt that her mother-in-law, Jeanine, had been very angry at her for many years because she blamed her granddaughter's drowning in the family pool on Sarah's negligence. Statements to this effect, made shortly after the child's death five years earlier, had driven a wedge between the two women. They remained cool and distant until Jeanine suffered a heart attack. Sarah's husband, Rod, who loved both his mother and his wife, felt it was time for the women to change their relationship. No longer willing to endure the tension, Sarah and Rod entered therapy to discuss the issues. Rod was torn between loyalty to his mother and to Sarah, and he carried his own burden of guilt because of his child's death. The in-laws were included in a subsequent session. As it progressed, Rod's mother claimed that she did not even remember making the remark. After a tense exchange, I discussed the grieving process and how the loss of a child affects the life of a family. Both women agreed that life was too short and that their love for Rod was more important than holding onto a grudge.

Death of a parent-in-law, the last stage in the individual life cycle, can also be devastating. Whether expected or unexpected, death can bring about grief issues that carry enormous impact through many subsequent years in the lives of survivors, especially if not resolved in a healthy way.

Active grieving for a spouse is a four-year process.

If you or an in-law has lost a spouse, remember that the active grieving for a spouse is a four-year process. Not all adjustments will take four years, but over the long run, it takes four years to arrive at a constant comfort level. Some events occur only once a year; Christmas, anniversaries, and holidays are very difficult times for in-laws who have lost a spouse. Other activities are done on a daily basis, such as grocery shopping, laundry, and the tasks of the daily routine. After doing these tasks four or five times, people usually become more comfortable doing them without the lost family member. For other events, like anniversaries and holidays, that take place on an annual basis, the survivor does not have as much *practice* in getting through them alone. It thus takes four years before the widow or widower learns how to get through these events without the loved one present.

It is helpful for in-laws to be aware that depression reaches its peak six months after the death. Americans are a death-denying society. We often feel that people should be *getting over it* in six months, rather than realizing that the height of depression following the loss of a spouse occurs after six months. Another important finding is that the second year after the loss of a spouse can often be more difficult than the first year. During the first year, the surviving in-law receives a lot of attention. By the second year, the supporting others have gotten back into their own routines, and the surviving spouse is left alone to try to adjust to the fact that the rest of his or her life will be lived without a significant other.

Grieving is a normal process, and drugs and alcohol can be very detrimental. *Just listening* to in-laws is important; you do not always have to *do*. Rules one, two, and three for helping grieving in-laws are: Listen, listen, and listen. Remember, all problems are not solvable; sometimes, in-laws just have to be heard.

When the surviving partner expects others to fill the lost space, difficult situations can arise for in-laws. A young couple came into therapy to discuss the wife's frustration with her 78-year-old father-in-law, who was recently widowed. She resented his desire to spend every minute of every weekend with the couple. "I don't even get to sleep in—he calls at 7:00 A.M. every Saturday to find out what we're doing," she said. "When we do anything with him, it's like we're going in slow motion—he has phlebitis and can't move very quickly. I thought I was marrying Mike, not his dad!" When the couple mentioned this in a therapy session, I pointed out that the father-in-law was in the early stages of grief.

He was probably feeling very vulnerable and needed predictability. The couple decided to plan events with him, marking them on his calendar three months in advance. They hoped this would take away his fear about being abandoned and would reassure him that they wanted to include him in their lives. The calendar device also took the couple off the hook from including him in everything they did. Gigi suggested that they give her father-in-law the option to cancel at the last minute, because she knew it was difficult for him to make plans. Her father-in-law needed closeness, but he also needed freedom to do the work of grieving. The couple and I discussed how the question for a newly widowed in-law is: "Where do I fit in?" We further explored how the father-in-law could be included in the family by setting limits but still keeping him empowered and involved.

As this case illustrates, spouses can feel quite angry about in-laws' demands. Pressure in this area can be eased by having a number of family members try to meet the unfilled roles and expectations left by the deceased in-law. James L. Framo, a well-known family therapist, says that, after a death of a spouse, children will have their loyalty tested when they are asked in subtle and not so subtle ways to help mother or dad out by doing some work around the house, driving to the doctor's office, or helping to get finances in order.

To help stabilize yourself or your in-laws after a death, I recommend that surviving spouses stay in their homes for a year before they make any decisions about selling their furniture or moving. They can then go through the early stages of grief in a familiar setting. Indeed, it would probably be better to stay for at least two years, to make reasonable decisions about future plans. It is difficult to see people go through this sadness and discouragement. However, in-laws should remember that surviving family members need to be *supported*, not *rescued*.

A widowed father-in-law can be especially challenging. The deceased spouse may have handled all social arrangements, and the man may not be used to making the social connections. In a study of widowhood, Trudy Anderson of East Texas State University at Texarkana found that widows have more primary ties with all kin than widowers do. Often, however, being widowed does not negatively impact close family ties—in fact, it strengthens ties with siblings, particularly sisters. Thus, a greater variety of kin are reported to be part of a woman's primary support network after the loss of a spouse.

Impact of Life Cycle Changes on In-Laws—Conclusion

In-law relationships will continue to change through the years—and those changes will be dependent on expected and unexpected life events, such as retirement, the empty nest, death, or divorce of an in-law. Roles will change as parents become experienced advisers and their children take on the adult roles of marriage, parenthood, and careers. As our population ages, in-laws will be challenged to keep their elderly members empowered, and to help them to deal with their declining physical, and sometimes mental, capabilities. At times, families may face the challenge of in-laws moving in—whether this means elderly parents-in-law moving in with their children, widowed in-laws moving in after the death of a spouse, or children-in-law moving in with the parents to get through hard times, save up to buy a house, or restart life after a divorce.

Roles will change as in-laws age.

Worksheet

Points for the family to discuss regarding the in-law family life cycle include:

1. In what ways can parents-in-law move into the role of experienced advisers?

2. Are family members having difficulty in accepting new roles?

3. Do we respect the contributions of the aging in-laws?

4. Has the family developed a clear idea of where older in-laws fit in?

5. Do the older in-laws have a life of their own?

6. How do the in-laws and children feel about living together?

7. Have other alternatives been considered if living together is not feasible?

8. Do we encourage our in-laws to be independent and functional?

9. Do we try to focus on in-law areas of competency by making affirming statements?

10. If in-laws are in grief over the death of a spouse, have we thought about ways we can support their four-year grieving process?

11. Do those living in the household understand that the height of depression comes six months after a death and that grieving is a normal process?

PART THREE

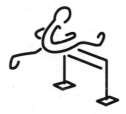

JUMPING IN-LAW HURDLES

7

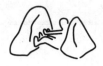

Between a Rock and a Hard Place—
Dealing with Divided Loyalties

What Does Family Loyalty Mean to the In-Law Relationship?

Loyalty to your birth family is natural. It gives a sense of closeness and affiliation toward those with whom you were raised and toward those who raised you. In order to love yourself, you must at least make peace and find connections of love with your birth family. If you do not love and respect those upon whom you were dependent in early life, it is difficult (if not impossible) to love yourself as an adult. How does this relate to in-laws? I have found through clinical experience that a spouse who develops increasing guilt over disloyalty to his or her parents may deal with the guilt by rejecting the spouse or the spouse's family. Take Jesse. When he was dating his girlfriend, he was very involved with her family. He even began to talk and act like they did. His family was from *the other side of the tracks.* After his marriage, he spent less time with his family and helped them out less. Instead, he bought clothes for trips and paid for the things he needed when he did things with his wife's family. Eventually, he started to feel guilty and unhappy; he noticed that his brothers and sisters did not have the kind of benefits that his siblings-in-law had. He felt torn: he could not give either family what they wanted and needed. Jesse began to withdraw from both his family and his wife's family.

In therapy, we began to talk about moderation. We explored how Jesse could moderate his visits to his family and to his wife's family. We discussed how he and his wife needed to form their own alliance and develop their own family traditions. Jesse and his wife then had a dialogue about his feelings on the issues. It was very enlightening to her, and they have begun to work on his problems of alienation.

To some degree, all relationships are burdened with each partner's unsettled accounts of loyalty to his or her family of origin. Loyalty to one's birth family is an often unrecognized force impacting in-law relationships. In *Invisible Loyalties,* Ivan Boszormenyi-Nagy and Geraldine Spark contend that loyalty cannot be measured, weighed, or seen. An invisible loyalty is a feeling one has for those who are important in one's life. Loyalty can cause people to behave toward in-laws in ways that may seem irrational to casual observers. In the context of a loyalty issue, however, the irrational behavior toward nonbiological family members begins to make sense. These same authors have identified a number of areas where there may be loyalty problems. I see the following areas as particularly sensitive in in-law relationships:

- **Intergenerational loyalty conflicts:** "Jack still subscribes to the caveat 'Don't trust anyone over 30,' and that includes his in-laws."

- **Couple vs. in-law loyalty:** "I want to build holiday traditions with our own new family, but Mary insists that we divide our holidays between our respective in-laws."

- **Loyalty obligations of spouse:** "Ever since Lucy's mom died, her dad expects Lucy to take dinner over every night."

- **Disloyalty to self:** "Because my sister-in-law and my husband stand to inherit the house equally, I have to endure her insults and feel I have compromised my self-respect."

To be able to grow spiritually and emotionally, you need to recognize and deal with the invisible bonds originating from your formative period of growth. Otherwise, you are apt to live them out as repetitious patterns in all your future relationships. Growth and change on the part of one family member can mean personal loss and relationship imbalance for another. The task is then to put the issues where they belong *in the early part of a new relationship*. Parents and siblings can acknowledge the change of relationship with their family members as they integrate a new in-law into the family system, all the while honoring the fact that loyalty to the birth family is a powerful influence. Over time, positive in-law loyalties can also develop.

Loyalty to the birth family is a powerful influence.

Family members may find it useful to identify whether they are experiencing loyalty *pulls*. In-law pulls say, "Hey, I'm not going to treat your mother any better than you treat my mother." Usually, this feeling is kept well below consciousness. It can be seen when a new member comes into the family, gets very involved with the in-laws, and then feels guilty: "What about my sister? What about my parents? How often are they going to see us?"

One young man, Irving, told me that when he and his wife, Miriam, went to their home state to visit their parents, they tended to spend more time with Miriam's parents, because it was easier for her to deal with the couple's children at her folks' house. Irving let the arrangement stand for several years, but then started to feel guilty and unhappy about his own parents. He finally demanded that they spend equal amounts of time with his parents. Miriam was not happy about this change; she had sisters and wanted to spend some time with them. The couple worked out their problem by visiting jointly with each set of parents and then spending some time separately with their own parents, so they were not together for the entire visit. In that way, loyalty issues did not become a big problem.

Every married couple belongs to three families—their own, and those of both sets of parents. When their parents-in-law have divorced and remarried, the number of family units to which the couple must establish loyalty expands dramatically. If the young family is to establish a strong family unit of its own, the children must inevitably realign their loyalties,

Every married couple belongs to three families.

placing their own newly established marriage before loyalty to their parents' families.

Realigning Loyalties between Parents-in-Law and the New Family

Be careful that you do not unwittingly cause in-law divisions by going to your in-laws for emotional support in disputes with your partner. Abraham Lincoln said it best: *A house divided against itself cannot stand.* In-law divisions are especially difficult if one partner dislikes an in-law to the point that he or she refuses to have contact with the in-law, thus forcing the other partner to choose between the in-law family and the spouse. This happened in the following case.

Over the years, Susan, a 35-year-old stockbroker, had a history of hurt feelings, slights, and general disagreements with the wife of her brother. She put up with what she considered to be plain jealousy on the part of her sister-in-law in order to maintain a good relationship with her brother and to avoid the heartbreak that she knew a family rift would cause her mother and father. A few months before Susan came to therapy, she had fallen in love and had plans to marry Sam, who was also a stockbroker. When Sam began to come to family gatherings, he observed and commented on how rudely Susan was treated by her sister-in-law. At first, Susan encouraged Sam's observations and felt vindicated after several years of abuse by her sister-in-law. But later, Susan paid a consequence for Sam's support. After he gave Susan a diamond engagement ring and Susan reported the sister-in-law's comment on the small size of the ring, Sam said that now his future sister-in-law had insulted him once too often and, as a matter of pride, he would not be in the same room with her again.

Susan was devastated when Sam refused to join her family for the upcoming Thanksgiving and Christmas holidays. In order to be with him, Susan arranged to spend the holidays with friends rather than her family.

In therapy sessions, Susan was shocked and surprised to see how she had contributed to the family schism by not dealing with her sister-in-law in the early stages of their relationship and by forming an alliance with Sam, who did not have her loyalty toward the family.

Susan and I spoke about the amount of energy it would take to realign those relationships. She did not feel ready to confront Sam at this time with her need to deal with her own in-law problems; she felt that approach might spoil their engagement and marriage. As a result of this decision, Susan will go into her marriage with a number of built-in in-law problems. I told Susan that I respect her decision and that I will be available to counsel with her when and if she needs help in dealing with her in-law problems.

Some in-laws stay neutral, some in-laws are totally supportive, and some in-laws will be there for you at one time and in someone else's corner at another time. Loyalty issues can be very tricky when loyalty to parents must be weighed against loyalty to a spouse. The climate can change quickly from supportive to combative. When police are called to break up domestic disputes, they may enter the house to try to work with the dispute, and have the family suddenly turn against them in a show of the power of family loyalty. If you are interested in keeping peace in your family, do not back people into corners, ask them to pick sides, or choose one loyalty or another. Loyalty can turn hot and cold, depending on the mood of the person. Suppose you come to town for a week to visit your in-laws. An argument breaks out, and one in-law sides with you, against the rest. When you leave, the in-law may be left to clean up the pieces or to try to deal with the in-laws that he or she has sided against.

The climate can change quickly from supportive to combative.

One of the sad things I see in therapy is a client's decision to actually give up his or her biological family for a spouse. I had one case where the spouse demanded that the wife choose—him or her family. She made the decision that, to keep peace, she would agree to see her family only once a year. This was a conscious, spoken decision, but other people must give up families because of geographical moves or refusals to visit or associate with them. Lack of acceptance of a spouse or family, or the desire of a spouse to spend time on his or her own activities, without considering what the mate might desire, can cause this separation.

Types of In-Law Family Loyalty

There are powerful gender connections between mothers and sons and between fathers and daughters. In their study of father–daughter relationships, Barbara Goulter and Joan Minninger discuss how these relationships can be replayed in the future; they can be determining factors in the health of an in-law relationship when the daughter eventually marries.

In-law relationships have some unwritten but extremely resolute loyalty rules. The first (and perhaps the strongest) is: "Nobody can take care of a son better than his mother." The corollary is: "For some women, nobody can be better than daddy." However, children of both sexes seem to feel closer to their mothers than to their fathers. In her study of blue-collar families, Mirra Komarovsky found that not only are the wives closer to their mothers than to their fathers, but the husbands were also closer to their mothers.

The relationship between the parents-in-law and their other children is another variable. Some parents may have to juggle or balance the needs of the biological children against the needs of sons- or daughters-in-law. Priss, the mother of four children, described her difficulty after two of her children were married. She had two in-laws, two dependent children at home, and two married children to deal with. "It's a real juggling act remembering everybody's birthday, deciding how much money to spend on everyone, and balancing how much time I spend with each," she said. Priss found that sometimes her married children were angry because they felt that the children who were still at home were getting more things than they ever got in their lives. "I think it impacts our in-law relationships at times," said Priss, "because the in-laws are naturally sympathetic toward their spouses. I have to say, 'That was then and this is now.' My husband and I have more resources now than we did when our older children were young, and we're just dealing with life the way it comes. I'm sorry my oldest son didn't get a bike until he was 14. But I don't see why that means that our youngest children shouldn't have things in their life." I reminded her of the saying, "Whoever said life would be fair?"

He Is My Son—Mother/Son Loyalty Pulls

The relationship between sons and mothers can be fraught with potential for problems. Diane stated that her mother-in-law had a stranglehold over her husband, Antonio, who laughed and said it was ridiculous. Diane added that she saw little need to spend time with birth families, now that she was married and had a family of her own. In discussing her family of origin, Diane stated that her father had never been home and had always done anything he wanted to do, but her mother was a slave to the family. Diane had decided not to follow in her mother's footsteps. With Antonio visiting his family all the time, Diane feared that she was becoming like her mother. The time Antonio was spending with his mother and siblings forced her to be alone to run the house, as her mother had. Further discussion revealed that her father, since divorcing her mother, had moved back in with his own mother. The couple resolved this issue by deciding to respect each other's needs. Antonio agreed to help more around the house so Diane could have some free time, and to schedule some couple's time as well. Diane agreed not to get upset about time he spent with his family, as free time was at the discretion of the user.

Another frustrated daughter-in-law, Margaret, a 26-year-old filmmaker, called me and complained that her mother-in-law was making too many demands on her husband's time. Margaret had recently married Lou, a 27-year-old sales representative. Lou's father had died of a heart attack one year previously, and because Lou was an only child, his mother, Patrice, was highly dependent on him and asked him to drive her everywhere. Margaret, the oldest of three daughters, resented the demands made on Lou.

Prior to the marriage, Margaret had enjoyed her future mother-in-law and had spent a good deal of time just hanging out with her, because her future husband lived at home. After the marriage, the couple bought a small home 30 miles away from Patrice. When the couple returned from their honeymoon, they waited several days to contact her. Within the week, the mother-in-law telephoned her son at his office, demanding to know why he had not contacted her and wanting to know when they were coming to visit. The couple went over to Patrice's house the next evening and, as Margaret put it, "All hell broke loose." Patrice let it be known that she expected Lou to take a vacation day from work and take her to the doctor. As the dutiful son of a widowed mother, Lou agreed to do it, but also warned her that Margaret would probably be angry that he had taken the day off. Patrice said to her daughter-in-law, "Lou knows you well. I can see by your face you don't like the idea."

Her mother-in-law had to realize that life goes on.

When the couple left the mother-in-law's house, Margaret blew up and told Lou that she had married him and not his mother. She further stated that Lou's mother needed to realize that Lou was someone else's husband now—and not his mother's boy. Lou became defensive and said that Margaret had to consider that his mother was dealing with his father's death. Margaret said that since it had been one year since the death, her mother-in-law had to realize that life goes on.

When Margaret telephoned me, the couple had not spoken for three days. I suggested that we have a joint session with Lou's mother. In the session, Patrice acknowledged her dependence, and Lou expressed his torn loyalties. On hearing Margaret's expression of distress at the situation, Patrice said, "Hey, he's my son. He belonged to me long before you even met, and I think I have a right to his help." Lou was aghast at his mother's expectations; he had felt he was only temporarily trying to ease the transition after the death of his father. Margaret acknowledged her mother-in-law's needs, but said she felt she had never been accepted in the first place as Lou's wife.

Margaret, Lou, and Patrice are caught in what Emily Martinsen and Joyce Bolender describe in their book, *The Troublesome Triangle*. The triangle is formed by a son, mother-in-law, and wife.

As grown-ups, certain kinds of behavior can block us if we do not give them up. Nurturing is not a one-sided activity. Margaret's mother-in-law wants help from Lou, but Lou is also getting things from his mother. To keep the relationship straight, Lou needs to continue to make verbal and physical gestures toward his mother that put him in a loving, responsible adult position while recognizing his responsibilities to his wife and family as well as his responsibilities toward his mother. When his mother makes an unreasonable request, Lou needs to be able to say no as an independent adult and not blame his wife or family that he is not able to spend more time with his mother. In this way, his wife and his mother might develop an adult friendship relationship because neither will blame the other for demands on Lou's time.

Nurturing is not a one-sided activity.

Because men, on average, die at an earlier age than women, many mothers-in-law are left without their husband's companionship. The son may possibly be drawn closer to his mother. Often, the son looks to his wife, the daughter-in-law, to help with the mother. But what if the daughter-in-law pulls out of the relationship? Will the son then come forward and take care of the mother, or will the mother be left out in the cold?

One client, Phoebe, said to me, "I constantly nag my husband to see his mother. I don't understand the fact that he can feel comfortable not seeing her for weeks at a time. I don't know whether it is because he counts on me to call her weekly, or because he really is that callous toward her. It scares me, because I wonder what he would do if I had physical problems. Would he take care of me or would he ignore me like he does his mother?"

I suggested that Phoebe might be enabling her husband, Winston, to not connect with his mother, because he knows she will. Phoebe decided to talk to Winston about her concern over his lack of connection with his mother. She said he was quite sheepish when she told him that, as the daughter-in-law, she felt concerned that she had to make all the contacts with his mother. She made a deal with Winston: Every other week, he would contact his mother and during the alternating weeks, she would contact her mother-in-law. She suggested further that, at least once a month, he could do something with his mother apart from her. Phoebe told Winston that if he decided not to do this, she would only contact his mother twice a month, for that is what she felt comfortable doing. Since Phoebe set that schedule, she has felt less burdened about getting together with her mother-in-law. Winston sometimes misses a week or two, but is now starting to have more meaningful contact with his mother.

Daddy's Girl—Father/Daughter Loyalty Pulls

Fathers can often wield too much power in their daughters' lives. A husband may have to live up to a feeling that his father-in-law is always right. There can also be a complementary role division: When father is hero, husband is failure; when husband is hero, father is failure. This was the case with the following family.

Although Patty's husband, Nathan, worked hard as a high-tech executive, he was often told by Patty that he was an ignorant man who could never live up to her father. Nathan, who was a teetotaler, could never figure out what his alcoholic father-in-law had achieved that he must *live up to*. Patty and Nathan's daughter, Amanda, seeing her father as a failure, picked an overachiever, Ronald, as a spouse, in order to fulfill what she saw as her mother's expectations of a man. Although Ronald was a highly successful executive, Patty resented her son-in-law, out of continued loyalty to her father. Patty even commented to Ronald that, when he had children, he would realize that no one is ever good enough for one's children.

Another client, Fay, had always been close to her dad, who was her swimming coach and always attended her meets. When Fay met Burt, she gave up her hopes of being an Olympic champion and dropped off the team.

Daddy became irate. He was the power in the family to whom everyone deferred. He could do no wrong, even when he walked out on the family to live with another woman. Later, to help Fay and Burt deal with marital problems, we had a family-of-origin session that included the entire extended family. As we looked at the family history, Fay's father admitted it was no coincidence that he walked out on the family when Fay left. "Without my little girl to take care of, there was no reason to hang around."

Dealing with In-Law Family Secrets and Myths

Most families have a skeleton or two in the closet, and keeping them there is, within limits, functional. Family secrets can serve to protect the self-esteem of the family members. Family secrets become a problem when they undermine mutual trust, inhibit dialogue, and distort reality in such a way that family adaptability and development become restricted." According to well-known family therapist James L. Framo, in the not-too-distant past, these secrets primarily revolved around abortion, homosexuality, illegitimate children, past marriages, and sexual peccadillos. Today, those family secrets are viewed as relatively mild compared to topics such as former drug abuse, alcoholism, imprisonment, incest, and rape, which are now the taboo subjects that form the base of the secrets held by families. According to Framo, the keeping of family secrets is a form of collective denial that is not necessarily pathological.

Most families have a skeleton or two in the closet.

One of the twists attached to family secrets is that new in-laws can instantly begin to believe that the problem concerns them rather than some past family history or family secret. There may be anger or touchiness around sensitive subjects like abortion because someone in the family has had an abortion. The in-law may not understand this, having no idea that the topic is so close to home. The unsuspecting in-law might say something critical or express very unwholesome attitudes that might have been softened if there was any realization that the subject was a family problem.

Family secrets need to be evaluated on an individual basis: Does an in-law need to be aware of a secret that is in the family? I had a client, Kate, who, in the past, had had an affair. She was currently married, and she and her husband had made an agreement that they would not tell her in-laws about the affair. They had resolved it together in therapy, and they felt that the in-laws, particularly the mother-in-law, would not be able to deal with this information. Kate's past relationship would be beyond her parents-in-law's comprehension of what was proper and acceptable behavior, and her present relationship with her in-laws would be permanently marred.

Is the secret long past? Is it impacting the family at this time, or could it impact the family in the future? What would be the purpose of telling the secret? Would knowing the secret hurt others? Whose secret is it to tell? Remember, opening up secrets must be age-appropriate; children may not be ready to hear secrets about affairs or sexuality. However, if a child-molesting in-law is part of a family or abuse is present, the other family members should always be told in order to protect their children.

Many behaviors can be difficult for in-laws to accept. However, physical abuse on an ongoing basis can be a different matter. If kept private and secret, the abuse often continues. Alcoholism, if still a secret, ought to be brought into the open in any family. (More on these topics in Chapter 12.)

Roger, a 43-year-old man in therapy, was a married man who had a problem of looking in people's windows—he was a *peeping Tom*. The couple decided to tell Roger's parents because they wondered whether there was any family history of sexual problems. Indeed, it turned out that Roger's father had had a problem with pornography and with his sexuality. That information opened up the whole family to look at its history of sexual behavior. Within the course of therapy, it was revealed that Roger's wife had been sexually molested by her father. Roger and his wife and the in-laws wanted to have the whole system exposed and dealt with, so that the secrets were not passed on to the next generation.

Avoid jumping quickly into a decision to expose secrets. The secret may have been kept for years, or generations. There is no hurry to tell it. The possible consequences should be given careful thought. If you are going to reveal a big family secret, you might plan ahead for it. Which of the in-laws should do the confronting, where it should be done, when, and why? If the secret is alcoholism, you might want to do an alcohol intervention and have a professional present. If the secret is incest, you might want to seek professional help or have a therapist present. A rule of thumb is: When things are difficult, it is helpful to enlarge the system by finding supportive people who can be there. People need to have a time to express their opinions and attitudes about the secret in a controlled and reciprocal manner.

When things are difficult, it is helpful to enlarge the system.

Regarding personal in-law secrets, you will want to think about how much an in-law secret blocks you as an individual. What price are you paying to keep your in-law secret from the rest of the family? Does holding your secret keep your in-laws from knowing who you really are as a person and from the honest relationship that you would like to have with them? Only you, as an in-law, can make this decision.

Although some therapists believe family secrets should not be unearthed, it is my experience that the majority of family members often either already know the secret or know that there is a skeleton in the closet.

Keeping the secret under wraps only diminishes the self-esteem of the entire family. Evan Imber-Black, Professor and Director of Family and Group Studies at New York's Albert Einstein College of Medicine, states in her book, *Secrets in Families and Family Therapy:* "Opening certain secrets may be profoundly healing for individuals and relationships, while opening other secrets may put people in jeopardy, particularly where issues of physical safety are concerned. And then there are secrets that hold the potential of both reconciliation and division, with no guarantees of which will pertain."

Opening certain secrets may be profoundly healing.

Such was the case for May, a botanist. When she and her husband met her sister-in-law's new boyfriend, they became suspicious over his reluctance to share any information about his background, his family, or even his job. "He seemed to have dropped from a void, and we worried about my sister-in-law getting in over her head with a man who clearly was hiding his past," said May. The couple hired a private investigator to get some rough information on the man, and it turned out that he was a member of the IRA (Irish Republican Army) and was in the United States illegally. Unfortunately for him, May's investigation tipped off the authorities and the boyfriend was soon extradited to Ireland. "My sister-in-law still hasn't forgiven us," May said.

If you talk to friends and associates in a general way about family secrets, you will find that most secrets are not unique to your family. Many families have similar bones in their closets. However, a caveat is required here: In some instances, it may not be wise or appropriate for you, as an in-law, to press for family secrets. Things may come out over time, and pressing for information may backfire on you—as was the case with May.

Restrain any tendency to pry into changes of mood or symptoms of problems that you observe in an in-law couple. Pressing for reasons, or offering to help may alienate you, the in-law, rather than resolve the problems.

There are functional and dysfunctional in-law secrets.

John Bradshaw, in *Family Secrets: What You Don't Know Can Hurt You*, makes the point that all families have secrets, and there are functional in-law secrets and dysfunctional in-law secrets. Do not take a polarized view of in-law relationships. Each family is unique within itself. High functioning in-law families are working on solving these problems within two or three weeks. Low functioning in-law families kick their problems under the rug and never talk about them.

Do Not Poison the Well

Be careful that you do not poison the well by making negative comments about your spouse to your siblings or parents, especially if they cannot keep a secret. When a spouse learns that the in-laws know too much about him or her, or know the wrong things, he or she may decline to get together with the in-laws, which will naturally cut down on the time you are able to spend with your family. "I am sorry that I told my mother that Jed had smoked pot before we got married," said Elaine. "The other day she asked him to give my kid brother, his brother-in-law, a lecture on the woes of drug using. Jed was really embarrassed that his in-laws thought he was a drug user."

As an in-law, it may be helpful to make the distinction between privacy and secrecy. Privacy is a human right. Through technology and intense media coverage of even local events, we have lost a certain amount of privacy in our culture.

Privacy is a human right.

Of course, some secrets should be held by adults and not shared with children, while others, such as surprise birthday parties, or Christmas or anniversary presents are traditionally fun secrets, that, to the frustration of in-laws, are often difficult for children to keep. Recently, my three-year-old granddaughter slipped away with my son-in-law while we were out to dinner. They were gone for about 20 minutes. When my granddaughter came back, she had a big grin on her face and she reached into her pocket and pulled out a little packet of birthday candles. The next day was my birthday, and since her daddy had told her it was a secret, she was very pleased to show what her secret was.

Boundaries with the Extended Family

Some in-laws are very needy, and their demands on others require a great deal of patience. These in-laws are referred to as *high maintenance*. If you let them in a little bit, they want in all the way. Their actions and neediness may make you move away—far away. With these in-laws, you might consider setting firm limits about what you will and will not do for them, to protect against their wanting more of you than you can give. Such was the case with the Jones family. Vanessa's husband's uncle popped in for a surprise visit, with his daughter and son-in-law and their two children in tow, when her husband was out of town. "It was wonderful to see him, we had a nice chat, and as the evening wore on, my uncle-in-law did not make any moves to leave, so I suggested that they stay for dinner," she said. They began hinting about how expensive Los Angeles hotels were, and it became clear that they were hoping that Vanessa would be able to put them up for the evening. As a full-time nurse, Vanessa had to be at work at 5:00 A.M. the next morning, and putting up her uncle-in-law and family was just not something she was prepared to do. She told them about a fairly inexpensive motel close to her home, but her uncle-in-law felt that it was too expensive, and they went to a Motel 6 outside the city.

Saying No to In-Laws

Practice saying, "No, No, No."

Nancy Reagan started the *Just Say No* trend. It is not always easy to say no to your in-laws. In fact, most of us do not ever just say no to anyone. Sometimes, I recommend that clients practice saying, "No. No. No." For many, it is a new activity. Others, however, say no before they even hear the question. You may need to ask those in-laws if they will at least listen to the whole story before they make a judgment.

For a time, my sister was living in Zimbabwe, Africa. She said people in Zimbabwe hate to say no. In fact, rather than saying no to anyone, they say, "Yes, I can't do that." Does that sound like anyone you know?

Heading the list of problem in-laws are people who let things go, never say what they are planning on doing, or never give any notice that they are coming to dinner or will spend a holiday with an in-law. They do not treat in-laws with the level of respect that they would give a friend. They count on others' finding it difficult to tell family members *no*. In the long run, their behavior makes for a strained relationship.

Make a special effort to be clear with your in-laws about what you will and will not do. Also, deliver only your own opinion and let people know that, if they want to know what your spouse thinks, they will have to ask your spouse themselves. Often, it is harder for a biological child to say no to family members than it is for an in-law. The in-law ends up getting labeled as the one who is always saying no to activities when actually the biological child is using the spouse to keep the family at bay.

All in-laws need to set limits on the family. Indeed, limits are essential in order to be involved with your family and still have a happy marital relationship and happy in-law relationships. Limit setting can be difficult. Initially, the limits you set may be too firm or too loose, but only by setting some limits can you know what will be comfortable for both you and your in-laws. This is a tricky situation because a number of people are involved, but it is worth working on. In-laws are long-term relations, and learning to set limits and enjoy your relationship with them can be an important and rewarding part of your life.

If you are having difficulty setting limits I would suggest that you and your partner or spouse chart out your expectations. Use the following format as a model:

What in-laws would I like to see?	How often would I like to see these in-laws?	What number of hours would I like to spend with these in-laws?	What activities would I like to do with these in-laws?
Sister-in-law	Once a month	4–6	Golf or tennis
_____	_____	_____	_____
_____	_____	_____	_____
_____	_____	_____	_____
_____	_____	_____	_____
_____	_____	_____	_____

Have your spouse or partner go through this same activity. Compare your expectations and then align any divergence on the frequency and number of hours that you would like to spend with in-laws. Be specific: Write *mother-in-law, father-in-law, brother-in-law, sister-in-law,* so that you are not saying you would like to spend time with *parents-in-law.*

When you finish this activity, compare your chart with your spouse's. In this way, your wishes are clear and in the open, and you can negotiate a difference in opinion about spending time with in-laws. You might agree that one spouse can spend some time with certain in-laws without the other spouse being involved, but the separate visiting times should not include special holidays and vacation. Those are times when a spouse will resent the other spouse's absence. Consider involving other family members in the chart-making activity. Understanding their expectations can also be helpful.

Dealing with Divided In-Law Loyalties—Overview

Only a foolish in-law would dive into the relationship head first.

Until you start forming alliances with your new in-laws, your primary connection with in-laws is through your partner. Consider the relationship as untested waters. You would not consider diving head-first into an unexplored lake or pond, and only a foolish in-law dives into the relationship without first testing it for unexposed obstacles. Your approach can be the difference in being seen as an intruder, a scapegoat, or a welcomed guest. Tread lightly, and develop relationships slowly. Let your experiences with your new in-laws develop naturally and in their own time.

For the most part, in-laws desire friends, not foes. Friends, if they are close enough, do occasionally step harmlessly on each other's toes. If you expect this to happen, view it as par for the course rather than as a strain on in-law loyalty. With some in-laws, you will have problems. Be prepared to invest more energy in making those relationships work, especially if your partner has strong loyalty connections to his or her mother, father, or siblings. Do not try to step into the middle of these intensely loyal relationships. Instead, develop your own relationship with these in-laws, separate from your partner's.

Following are some questions that will help you think about how you and your in-laws align loyalty.

Worksheet

1. Do you feel tension regarding the loyalty you have for your biological parents versus your in-laws?

2. What kinds of loyalty issues do you think you might encounter in relationships with your biological family, in-laws, and nuclear family?

3. What kind of in-law boundaries do you maintain? (Can your spouse talk to the in-laws about your marital arguments?)

4. In what ways can you understand and accept your spouse's loyalty to his or her family of origin (your in-laws)?

5. Do you have family secrets that are kept from the in-laws? How will you handle them and still maintain family loyalty?

6. Are there differences between your expectations of boundaries and your in-laws' expectations?

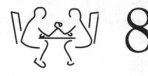 8

Who's the Boss? The Struggle for Power

Who Has the Power?

Who has the power for change in the family?

If you want to make changes that involve your in-laws, you have to identify who has the power in the relationship. In Physics 101, we all learned that any large object can be moved if you have a lever and can find the fulcrum or the center point needed to move it. If you imagine a seesaw, with you and your in-law going up and down on opposite ends, you can picture how you need to move the balance of that relationship to produce change. First, you must find out where the center point is and who has the power for change in the family.

At a recent international conference of family therapists, held in Guadalajara, Mexico, I gave a presentation about my work with in-laws and in-law therapy. During the discussion, an Ethiopian woman said that mothers are very close to their sons in Ethiopia, and tend to baby them and give them whatever they want and desire. When she gave further details, we came to the conclusion that there are good reasons for this in-law dynamic. In her part of Ethiopia, men still retain the dominance and the power to control resources. Therefore, it behooves the mother to stay closely connected and involved with her son, because he is the person who will take care of her and protect her as she ages. Women tend to outlive men, so he will probably support her beyond the death of her husband; thus, her son has the power in the relationship.

When you are looking at power for change, you have to understand the economics and the culture you are dealing with. You would not ask an Ethiopian woman to stand up and confront her male in-laws, because the power lies with her son. Any confrontation would have to be led by the biological male who would be most likely to advocate change in the family.

Balancing In-Law Expectations

Sometimes, by expecting too much loyalty from our children, we destroy the possibility of a relationship with our in-laws. Frieda's daughter had leukemia, and Frieda worked very hard with her as she went through treatments. The pain of the whole process ultimately destroyed Frieda's marriage, and she said, "I feel that [the daughter] owes me for a lost life that I had because of all the hours I spent taking care of her, and now I have a son-in-law who doesn't want to spend a lot of time with me at my house." Frieda felt that her son-in-law had broken the bond between her and her daughter.

Through therapy, Frieda realized that the bond she had with her daughter was not necessarily healthy. She felt her daughter owed her a bond of debt. The daughter also felt it and, in a therapy session, cried and said that she could never repay her mother for her life, but her mother just expected more than she could give.

Meeting In-Law Emotional Needs

You may say, "I can't even meet my own emotional needs; how would I go about meeting my in-law's?" As human beings, we need certain things, and one of them is human contact. We also need to be cared for, loved, and assured that we are valued and are an important part of our family's world. All of us want to be heard, listened to, not overlooked,

The better you know your in-laws as individuals, the better you will know what it is that they are trying to get from you.

and accepted, even in our eccentricities and problems. So, the better you know your in-laws as individuals, the better you will know what it is that they are trying to get from you. What kind of attention do they want? Are they willing to take negative attention, rather than no attention at all? Would acknowledgment of them help to move from negative attention toward positive attention?

What are your own emotional needs? What do you need from your in-laws? Does your agenda need time alone, while their agenda needs time together? How can you negotiate their needs and still meet your own needs? Go down the list: "What is it I want from my daughter-in-law (or mother-in-law)? What do I want from my son-in-law (or father-in-law)? What do I want from my sibling-in-law?" Then ask yourself, "What does each of these individuals want from me?"

Do this activity with your spouse or partner and compare your ideas on what biological family members need from you, and what your in-laws need from you.

Blaming Your Spouse for In-Law Problems

A young professional couple, Ted and Mindy, came to therapy in the wake of a disastrous week-long visit from Ted's parents. As Ted drove his departing parents to the airport, his mother stated that the next time they came, they would stay in a motel and would rent a car, because she felt that staying with Ted, Mindy, and their young son was just too confusing. Ted was hurt and Mindy was angry. In discussing the history of the family with the young couple, Ted said that he had always been very close to his dad. Often, that closeness excluded his mother. Initially, his mother welcomed Mindy into the family. With Mindy taking her son's attention, she foresaw more time to spend with her husband—time that he was now spending with their son. Mindy, however, did not see Ted's dad as a threat. She encouraged Ted to spend as much time with his father as possible while she kept busy with her own activities. Mindy saw her mother-in-law as a couch potato who lacked initiative and ambition. Mindy's attitude helped to position Ted's mom as a nagging mother-in-law.

I felt it important to help the couple view the situation as an in-law problem, although it was obvious that Ted had been brought in to ease the tension and balance the power between Ted's mother and father.

Ted and Mindy decided that they would like to be able to have an enjoyable visit with both of Ted's parents. We sought to determine what an enjoyable visit would look like, and Ted said he was willing to give up some time with his father in order to include his mother. Mindy agreed to give up some of her community activities and spend time with Ted's parents during the next planned visit. We then discussed some of the goals for the visit. One was to keep the age hierarchy straight: to keep both Mom and Dad in the *experienced adviser role*, as grandparents and parents-in-law. We discussed elevating Mom by asking her opinions and getting her involved in planning joint activities. We also sought to avoid loyalty struggles by refraining from comparisons between Ted's mother and Mindy's mother, who is more active and lives in the same neighborhood. The couple was encouraged to accept Ted's mother as an individual and not look at her as strictly a mother-in-law or grandmother. We then discussed some ways to ease the tension. One was to plan activities each day as couples. Another was to get a baby-sitter for a weekend or overnight so the couples could take a trip together. All of these strategies helped Ted and Mindy see his parents—especially his mother—in a new light, and made for a more successful in-law relationship on subsequent visits.

Keep the age hierarchy straight.

Blaming Your In-Law for Spousal Problems

"It's Either Me or Them"

One of my clients, Florence, made this comment three or four times during the course of several weeks of therapy; she wanted her husband to make a choice between her and his family. When I asked her why she felt this choice had to be made, she said, "Well, it's either me or them. He

Giving love to a mother or father does not mean less love for a spouse.

can't have it both ways." My question was, "Why can't he have it both ways? Why can't he have a loving relationship with his parents and still have a loving relationship with you?" She said, "Because he does what they tell him to do, then he doesn't do what I want him to do." I said it is really not a matter of love or choosing, it is a matter of behavior. She agreed, and I suggested that the issue was not between her husband and his parents. It was a power issue between her and her husband—how they negotiated tasks and activities. I suggested to Florence that she needed to be more specific about what she wanted from her husband and to entertain the idea that these relationships are not mutually exclusive—a person can love his or her parents and still love the spouse. Giving love to a mother or father does not mean less love for a spouse, and the spouse who encourages love between the in-laws actually accumulates power in a very subtle way.

These are different kinds of love, and it is possible to maintain both of them intact; however, people need to learn to set boundaries, to let their partner know honestly what their needs and desires are, and to negotiate, as adults, what they require from relationships. If the husband understands what his wife requires, then he can go to his mother, father, or siblings and set limits with them on what he will and will not do.

In-Laws in the Middle

Many in-laws wind up in the middle of a problem between a couple.

Many in-laws wind up in the middle of a problem between a couple. Sometimes, they are not even aware that they have been roped in until it is too late. The good news is that these problems can sometimes be resolved without the actual presence of the in-law.

I had seen Nell, a clothing designer and mother of three-year-old Jessica, for one year in individual therapy before she told me that she wanted to leave her husband Kenneth for another man. Nell had not yet disclosed her feelings to her husband. I suggested to Nell that, before things went any further, we should ask Kenneth in to talk about the problem. Nell agreed, as long as she could tell Kenneth her plan in my office. The couple came to therapy several days later. Nell told Kenneth that she was in love with her old high school boyfriend, Lorin. Kenneth said he had suspected something, because Lorin had kept in touch with Nell since their marriage and in the last month had called her weekly from his home in Colorado. Kenneth, who loved Nell deeply, had been aware of Nell's friendship with Lorin, but they had agreed that their marriage would end it. Kenneth begged her not to leave him and their daughter Jessica.

After the session, Kenneth called Nell's mother, his mother-in-law, for emotional support. After her conversation with Kenneth, the mother called Nell and read her the riot act, saying that she was an embarrassment to the whole family. Nell hung up on her mother and refused to answer any subsequent calls or letters.

Because Nell would not respond, her mother began making frequent calls to the hospital where Kenneth was doing his residency. She demanded to know why Nell would not answer her calls. Kenneth discovered during one very emotional call that his mother-in-law was even threatening to go to court to try to win custody of Jessica. She said it sounded like he was at the hospital the majority of the time, leaving her granddaughter with an unfit parent. Kenneth just said, "Jessica is fine, and Nell is a good mother. I really can't talk now."

At the next therapy session, I discussed with Kenneth and Nell how they had drawn the mother-in-law into an *emotional triangle*, a very precarious situation because of its inherent instability as a relationship structure (we all remember the saying, *Two's company, three's a crowd*).

During our couple's therapy session, I drew a triangle on a large pad and we discussed the idea of emotional triangles and how, when the stress between Nell and her mother was too great, Nell's mother triangled in Kenneth by telephoning him at the hospital. However, I pointed out that Kenneth was responsible for the original triangle. He had contacted his mother-in-law to intercede in the stress between himself and Nell.

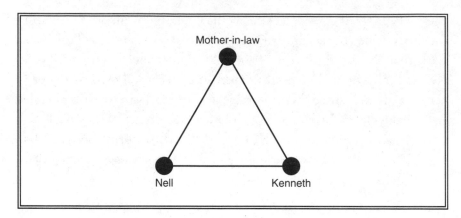

An Emotional Triangle

Kenneth then asked how to get out of this triangle. I suggested that he might respond in a different manner when talking to his mother-in-law, especially when she acted as though he was unable to take care of himself or his family, or when her mother told Nell that she was an embarrassment to the whole family.

Acknowledge the triangle of grandmother, grandchild, and parents.

Both Kenneth and Nell decided to respond by supplying information that would help the mother-in-law take on the role of a concerned grandparent. They felt that emphasizing the value of this role would help her decrease her involvement with the couple's problems. This response would acknowledge the triangle of grandmother, grandchild, and parents, which was of vital concern to all of the parties involved.

Because Kenneth was least caught up in the family emotional system, he agreed to make the first attempt at changing the family dynamics. Kenneth telephoned his mother-in-law that evening, while Nell was at book club. He told his mother-in-law that he and Nell knew that she was a very concerned grandparent. He told her about Jessica's day care and put Jessica on the line to say hello. He said that Nell was fine and that they were going to counseling, hopeful that things would work out. His mother-in-law was very responsive to the new triangle of parents, grandchild, and grandmother. Kenneth ended the conversation by saying that either he or Nell would call her the following Sunday and that it was better if he called her, as it was difficult to talk at the hospital. Kenneth also told his mother-in-law he would send her some of Jessica's artwork.

At the next therapy session, Kenneth said that, during the phone call, his mother-in-law was at first suspicious and a bit guarded, but after speaking with Jessica, she had melted like butter. She said she looked forward to hearing from them the following Sunday. I continued to counsel with the couple for several months. Nell decided that leaving her family for Lorin was too high a price to pay. Shortly thereafter, Kenneth finished his residency and the family moved to New Mexico. One year later, I received a Christmas card with a picture of the smiling faces of Kenneth, Nell, Jessica, and their new baby boy, Christopher.

Solving In-Law Conflicts

What do you want from your family or from your in-laws? What would you consider as functional ways to connect with your in-law family? You might want to look at where you are on the continuum of conflict → distance → cutoff, and then take a look at where you would like to be. We think of conflict as a negative term, but there are some positives about conflict. Healthy conflict in which you are able to bring up difficult issues can help you to work through relationships with your in-laws and can lead to stronger and better-understood interactions.

There are some positives about conflict.

Some clues to solving conflicts in in-law relationships are offered by Evelyn R. Duvall's survey of in-laws. Although this study is dated, it still provides some clues to major in-law disagreements. I believe these disagreements carry over to other problems of in-laws.

By asking people questions—"What was annoying about your in-laws?" "What did you disagree about?"—Duvall found four areas of major in-law disagreement:

1. **Inflexible:** *This is how things were done in my family.*

   "My husband told me that he thought it was important to hang the clothes out on the clothesline, because he agreed with his mother that it not only made them whiter but also killed any bacteria that may be on them. I said that if the clothes were hung that way, he and his mother would have to come and do the whole job, because I was working full-time and did not have the luxury of spending time hanging clothes outside. This was early in my marriage, and I have since found that this isn't the only issue that my mother-in-law is inflexible about. Some things I stand up for and others aren't worth my time and I just let them go."—Diana, 34, dental assistant

2. **Too permissive:** *My mother-in-law was very upset when I let her three-year-old granddaughter dig in the garden.*

   "My mother-in-law and I are very different regarding my children. She kept my husband in a walker until he was able to walk, because she didn't want him to get dirty. I on the other hand think that being involved in dirt is just one of life's activities that helps children to understand the difference between clean and dirty. She said, 'I can't believe you'd let her get that dirty.' And I said, 'Well, as long as she's having fun. They say earthworms are a good source of protein.'"—Miriam, 26, homemaker

3. **Differing views:** *My parents-in-law only had one child, my husband. According to them, they were always in control and made sure he never cried.*

   "Both my mother-in-law and father-in-law got very upset when I came to visit them. I remember sitting on the porch and having them glance askance at me while the baby cried. These behaviors were acceptable in my family, which maintained a more casual environment, but the behavior placed an imposition on the in-laws' more organized household. I realize we do have differing views but we learn to live and let live."—Claudia, 45, legal clerk

4. Pretentious: *My brother-in-law was critical of our family as we changed into casual clothes after Sunday services and his family stayed in formal dress the entire day.*

"My brother-in-law thought somehow his family was superior because they had better manners than my family. Every time he comes up with one of his pious comments, I realize that's just him and I try to concentrate on the many positive aspects of his personality."— Bonnie, 24, electrician

These are among the many possible styles that foster in-law disagreement, and none of them is necessarily wrong. People like to have their own positions affirmed. For example, one mother-in-law became extremely agitated with her daughter-in-law because she expected her to be the *family correspondent*, and she had not heard from the couple for several months. To deal with her anger, she sent a postcard to her daughter-in-law with the message, "I have polio." A week later she received a postcard in reply. Her daughter-in-law was asking, "Are you on a respirator?" Although these kinds of in-law struggles for recognition can seem amusing, they are at worst destructive and, at best, highly unproductive.

New in-laws entering a family can become unwitting participants in ongoing interpersonal issues between family members. "I know this family had some long-standing problems so why as an in-law should I get blamed for them? If I don't take the blame, I seem to get shut out." Monica McGoldrick identifies three unhealthy ways in which a couple may deal with their in-laws:

New in-laws entering a family can become unwitting participants in ongoing interpersonal issues between family members.

1. Conflict: "My father-in-law treats my husband like he's still a child and says rude things to him. It makes me angry and so when we're together, I give my father-in-law the cold shoulder. I'll turn and talk to my mother-in-law or my brother-in-law and I just answer my father-in-law with a one-word answer. I know that he knows that I don't like him, and frankly I'm glad."—Sherene, 42, retail manager

2. **Enmeshment:** "We're always over at my in-laws' house. We watch sports and games and eat pretzels and peanuts and party there. My in-laws expect us to spend every weekend with them unless we check in and tell them that we'll be doing otherwise. They also expect that we will spend all the holidays and vacations with them. So far, we've only been married a year and it seems to be going OK, but I have a feeling that at some point we're going to need to set limits on them, especially after we have children. I think it's going to be tough to tell them no."—Donna, 27, sales clerk

3. **Distance and emotional cutoff:** "I never had any problems with my in-laws, because I was smart enough to move 2,000 miles away. As far as I'm concerned, where family is concerned, the less the better."—Manfred, 40, bank manager

You will have to decide what you want your relationship with each person to look like.

McGoldrick explains that the ideal for a couple is being independent of their families while maintaining close and caring ties. As mentioned earlier in this book, you might want to think in terms of interdependence rather than independence. However, each family is made up of individuals, and you will have to decide what you want your relationship with each person to look like. There are some choices, and you can put some definition to the way your in-laws interact and how you would like to interact with them.

I believe that if you honor the age hierarchies, you will honor and respect your in-laws and will understand how to take proper action and deal with them in a functional way. If your instincts are guided toward love and respect, trust your instincts and follow them. Too many of us have learned not to trust our instincts. If your instincts follow in the purpose of harmony and love, you will find that you are using correct action toward changing your in-law relationship.

If your motive is to get your own way or to get some revenge on an in-law who has hurt your feelings, you probably will not want to trust your instincts. Instead, look at what the long-range consequences of revenge might be. Is it more important to get revenge or to promote peace and harmony in your life?

Getting Along with Other Parents-in-Law— Whose Problem Is It, Anyway?

Sometimes, you might find yourself feeling more loyal and obligated to an in-law's family than is warranted. Zelda, a retired bookkeeper, belonged to a theater arts group with whom she went to the symphony every Wednesday. Her daughter's mother-in-law hinted very boldly that she would like to be invited to join the group. "I have problems with this," said Zelda. "My group is composed of old friends—we have been running the group together for ten years." Zelda's daughter and son-in-law have told her that she does not have to include the in-laws in all of her activities. However, she still feels somewhat guilty about not doing it. Zelda might want to assess whose problem it is. The son-in-law and daughter do not care whether the in-laws are involved with one another, so Zelda needs to resolve this issue in her own mind and, while remaining courteous to the in-law, realize that her daughter's mother-in-law is not her responsibility.

Before jumping in or continuing to take the major responsibility for an in-law(s), consider this list of questions:

- Whose needs am I meeting, mine or my in-law's?

- Do I feel that helping my in-laws is a huge personal sacrifice for me as an in-law?

- Do I have the misconception that I am irreplaceable as an in-law caregiver and that others will not or cannot help?

- Do I sometimes resent helping my in-law(s)?

- Do I feel that I am doing another in-law's work or taking another family member's responsibility?

- Am I enabling other family members to avoid responsibility by being an overfunctioning in-law?

- Am I prepared to continue this in-law enabling behavior as a lifetime responsibility?

- What is the worst thing that can happen if I refuse to do the job and stop enabling?

- What is the best thing that can happen if I share the responsibility of caring for an in-law with my partner, family, church, and community?

Keepers of the Kin

Historically, women (more than men) are responsible for interpersonal and intrafamily relations. Sisters-in-law, as well as mothers-in-law, are frequently (and I think unfairly) criticized for failures in achieving harmony with the extended family. Sisters-in-law have an especially difficult harmonizing role because the term *sister-in-law* refers to several relationships that must be balanced: brother's wife, wife's sister, husband's sister, husband's brother's wife, and others more remotely related. In terms of sister-in-law relationships, the wife's sister is least often a problem, and the husband's sister is the most difficult.

Women can be seen as something of a family glue.

Women have a big responsibility for fostering family relationships. They can be seen as something of a family glue. Benjamin Franklin's old saying "My son is my son 'till he takes a wife, but by daughter's my daughter all the days of my life" has been around a long time—for good reason. I like to tell my clients that the reason a daughter's a daughter all of her life is because women traditionally have been in charge of the home, and many wives take responsibility for the relationship with their husbands' families as well as their own.

Women often say in therapy, "I told him that she's his mother, not mine." This addresses the fact that men often see their wives as keepers of the kin and even feel their wives should take care of the men's own biological mothers. Through the life span, these men have probably had difficulty setting limits and developing adult relationships with their mothers, and in some cases, siblings.

Why Is the Mother-in-Law Predominant in Family Power Issues?

As a mother-in-law, I am saddened when I hear people talk about how controlling or demanding their mother-in-law is. I find it particularly disturbing to hear this from other women. These women may someday be mothers-in-law themselves and will face the same prejudices and problems. Many women do not seem to be aware that scapegoating other women, including mothers-in-law, will come back to haunt them. Their children will hear them talking about their mother-in-law, and the children will carry on those same attitudes.

What is going on here? Why are women having these feelings about their mothers-in-law? If you are a female, it is in your best interest to really look at this situation so you can avoid the trap of either doing what your mother-in-law is doing or scapegoating your mother-in-law and dumping on her some issues that are really about someone else. Ask yourself, "Is this issue about my mother-in-law or is it about me?"

If mothers-in-law are a problem, we need to get to the root of what they are doing that is problematic in the family. It is time to stop passing along this *wicked mother-in-law* tradition. In my in-law research, I ask the question, "With which in-law do you have the most problems?" Mothers-in-law are consistently identified as the most problematic in-laws. I hope that through targeted interviews I can more extensively look into why this is the case. I have replicated the research of Evelyn R. Duvall, who surveyed more than 7,000 people to find out their views on

It is time to stop passing along this wicked mother-in-law tradition.

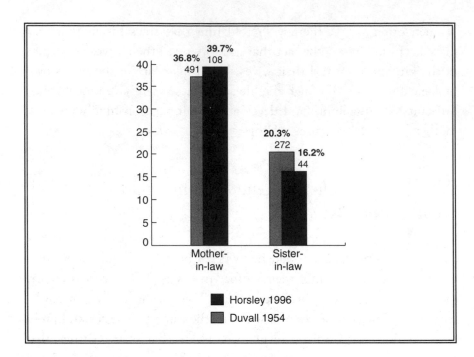

Horsley-Duval Bar Chart

in-laws. My preliminary findings strongly correlate with Duvall's work more than 40 years ago: the mother-in-law is most problematic, followed by the sister-in-law (husband's sister).

Why is the mother-in-law seen as most problematic? Paula J. Caplan, Assistant Professor of Psychology at the University of Toronto and an expert on mother–daughter relationships, sees mother-blaming as a way to keep the status quo and a way to avoid power shifts from men to women.

A few decades ago, during the height of the women's movement, an article was given to me by my supervisor at the University of Rochester School of Nursing. The gist was that *everyone needs a mother*, including mothers, and that the expectations we have of a mother are not possible to meet. Thus, being the ideal mother-in-law is also an impossible goal.

Although the mother's connection with the children is a natural result of the social structure, the mother–child bond has been criticized, rather than understood, by the mental health community as well as by the public. Mothers-in-law have been made the brunt of jokes and cruel comments. Instead of understanding the dynamics of the mother–child relationship, in-laws, and especially mothers-in-law, have been lampooned and avoided. Brothers-in-law and fathers-in-law are seen as less problematic. The most common complaints heard about brothers-in-law involve incompetency, immaturity, and irresponsibility. The most common complaints lodged against fathers-in-law center on meddling, nagging, and criticism. The father-in-law syndrome appears to feature ineffectuality and resistance to change; the mother-in-law is seen as interfering and demanding.

The mother–child bond has been criticized, rather than understood.

In-Law Bashing

Many in-laws engage in the not-so-fun game of in-law bashing—making in-laws the brunt of a continual stream of insults and put-downs. Often, a spouse will denigrate the parents-in-law in order to make his or her own parents look good in comparison. In-law bashing may affirm one's own parents in the short term, but, over the long term, it is destructive. In therapy, many clients engage in projecting onto the in-laws the anger they bear toward their own parents.

In-law bashing over the long term is destructive.

Nick and Tammy came to see me in order to discuss their increased hostility toward one another. The fights had escalated to the point of pushing and slapping. Frequently, their fights were about Tammy's close relationship with her mother and the fact that Nick's parents were never allowed to tend the couple's two-year-old daughter, Heidi. Nick and Tammy spent the majority of their family time, including holidays and vacations, with Tammy's parents and virtually ignored Nick's parents. For the first few years of their marriage, this arrangement had been fine with Nick. He had had a great deal of resentment toward his parents for what he described as an overly restrictive and sometimes physically abusive childhood. Cutting his parents out of his life, he felt, was nothing more than they deserved.

As Heidi got older, Nick began to see his little daughter's love for Tammy's parents and the delight it brought to Tammy. Nick began to long for a relationship with his parents that included Tammy and Heidi. When he approached Tammy with the idea of mending fences with his parents, Tammy was surprised and resistant. How did Nick know that Heidi would be safe with Nick's parents after what they had done to him? Nick quickly found himself defending his parents and talking up their good qualities. Tammy continued to react negatively. In retaliation, Nick began to criticize her parents and became more resistant to his in-laws. Unfortunately, in this circumstance, Tammy's in-law bashing had negative consequences in Nick's relationship with her parents.

When my own daughter married, my husband reminded me to encourage my daughter to visit her in-laws, saying, "You are only going to get treated as well by your sons-in-law as your daughters treat their mothers-in-law." It was very good advice, and I do not complain when my older daughter and her husband spend every other Christmas with his family. Indeed, I assume that, at some time, they will want to spend Christmas on their own and have their own family rituals.

Honesty, goodwill, and humor go a long way.

The goal is to *overcome* individual issues and dependency needs without overcoming the parents and in-laws. Nobody wants to be guilty of tossing out the baby with the bath water. Honesty, goodwill, and humor go a long way toward refining and defining expectations of these special relationships.

The In-Law Power Struggle—Overview

Although some observers might disagree, most in-law relationships are fraught with struggles for power—above and beyond the loyalty alliances: power to make things happen, power to make decisions about family activities, power to forge new bonds or sever old ones, power for change. If you are struggling to control your own life or your own destiny as an in-law, you might be caught up in a power struggle that you cannot win. Rather than trying to wrest power, you need to follow the natural lines. Instinctively, one would think that power in the family lies with the parents, but this is not always the case. The power for changing an uncomfortable situation may or may not be held in age hierarchies, but it is most often held by the biological family members. Sometimes, you can talk to in-laws directly about your problems, but your approach must be subtle; if you are not able to make quiet changes, you may have to bring in the *big guns*, which usually means your partner, or the person who biologically connects you to the in-laws. Then, you must carefully select the biological family member who has the ability to change the situation. One person does not hold the power to change all situations. Family members tend to have domains over which they control not only the pace, but the rules and the play. Calculate your moves carefully.

It is tempting for the men in the family to sit back, stay quiet, and let the women of the family "fight it out"; however, this is seldom productive, and the family tends to get stuck in place. Old gripes and annoyances are repeated on a regular basis. Unhealthy in-law situations can then become predictable: "That's just the way my mom is." People become written off or discounted when bad behavior is expected and accepted.

It is tempting for the men to sit back and let the women fight it out.

Following are some questions to help you identify where the power lies in your in-law relationships, and to clarify steps you might consider if you want to see change happen. I recommend that you start out small, and work through a specific, fairly benign in-law situation that you find uncomfortable. Once you have some successes under your belt, move forward to bigger problems.

Worksheet

1. Identify a situation where you would like change to occur.

2. Who in the family has the power for change in this situation? (Hint: Look at the biological family lines.) Approach that person directly and request change.

3. Look at your own family issues. Have you inadvertently let your spouse deal with them by reframing them as in-law issues?

4. Have you established limits, and are you able to say no to your in-laws?

5. Do you or your in-laws have an unacknowledged need for a *time-out?*

6. Do you engage in in-law bashing? Are you aware of the long-term risks of this behavior in terms of biological loyalty? (Your spouse may turn on you and yours.)

7. Do you blame your in-laws for spousal or partner problems? Do you blame your spouse or partner for in-law problems?

8. Do you allow your in-laws to have their personal space? Do you receive personal space from your in-laws?

9. Are you invalidating your in-laws' needs or desires?

10. Are you able to balance your biological family with your in-laws? Do you ever feel that you must give up your biological family for your in-laws, or vice versa?

11. Do you enable others to avoid responsibility for in-law relationships? Do you promote dependence or regressive behavior on the part of your in-laws by overfunctioning for them?

12. If you are caught in the middle between in-laws and your partner, what steps do you plan to take to extract yourself?

9

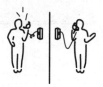

Can We Talk? Coping with Communication Problems

We all communicate all the time, whether we say anything or not. Often, what is left *unsaid* communicates more than the spoken word. Our body language can speak volumes. Arms folded over the chest is usually the position of someone who is trying to protect himself or herself. Clenched fists, tears, loud laughter—all send their own messages. Because we are always communicating, it seems prudent to learn how to communicate well with those around us, especially our in-laws.

Communication is a vague term. Couples come to therapy with the complaint that they cannot communicate with their in-laws. I tell them, "In the first place, you must realize that you are always communicating something. . . . If you are not speaking, that's communication. If you are not looking at someone, that's communication. If you leave the room, you are communicating something. The question is: How can you have the kind of communications with your in-laws that you would like to have?"

Often, what is left unsaid communicates more than the spoken word.

Identifying In-Law Feelings

Often, simple identification of your own feelings on issues can be useful in providing a groundwork for future communication and problem solving with your in-laws. Marriage counselors Gerald Weeks and Stephen Treat have observed that family members get locked into the idea that certain feelings should not be felt or expressed. If you endorse this idea, ask yourself how feelings were handled in your family: Which feelings were acceptable and not acceptable? How were different feelings expressed? Then ask your spouse or interested in-laws to do the same, and compare your in-law family with your family of origin.

The following questions are suggested by Weeks and Treat. Try to keep your answers simple (one or two words for each question).

- What was the predominant feeling in your family? Who set the mood?

- Which feelings were expressed most often, most intensely?

- Which feelings were not allowed?

- How were members punished when an unallowed feeling was expressed?

- What happened to the unexpressed feelings in the family?

- Who knew/did not know about how others felt?

It will be enlightening for you to compare your partner's or your in-law's answers with yours. Sharing the commonalities and differences will help to foster a healthy in-law relationship. Our feelings reflect who we are and how we view others. When we have access to our full feelings and can express them in constructive ways, we can strengthen or expand our repertoire of communication skills.

Respecting In-Law Communication Styles

Greer, a 40-year-old attorney, was confused by his father-in-law, who said, "Come on up. Come and be around us. Spend a lot of time with us." But when Greer and the family arrived, the father-in-law barked at the children or seemed angry and just disappeared. Verbally, he said, "Come." Nonverbally, he said, "Your children aren't behaving correctly and I wish you weren't here; get out of my hair." When Greer tried to talk to him, the father-in-law said, "I haven't seen you for a long time. I hope you're going to be up to visit me soon." I told this client that there are some people whose eye automatically goes to error and to what is wrong in any situation. When in-laws are around, these people communicate an indictment of others' errors on a constant basis. They look for what is missing in the family picture rather than enjoying the fact that the in-laws are around and are involved with them.

Stop and think for a moment: What are you communicating to your in-laws? Are you saying one thing and doing another? Saying *Please come* and then behaving in bad ways? Or, are you saying *Stay away* and, when they do not come, feeling angry about it? What can you do to make your physical behavior more congruent with your verbal messages?

An Open Ear

In *The Lost Art of Listening*, Michael P. Nichols states that one of the biggest problems he sees in our society today is the fact that people do not listen. Not only do they not listen to others, but they do not listen to themselves. Nichols goes on to make some important points about listening. I have adapted them to listening to in-laws.

One of the biggest problems in our society is that people do not listen.

- Listening to in-laws is an active endeavor when, for a few moments, we suspend judgment.

- Most in-laws won't pay attention to your point of view until they think that you have heard theirs. You can give your in-laws the gift of understanding by listening with a minimum of defensiveness, criticism, or impatience.

- Simple failure to acknowledge what an in-law says leads to a great deal of in-law friction.

- Wise is the in-law who gives support but not advice.

- In-laws who learn to listen to each other with understanding and tolerance may find that they do not need to change each other.

- If we want the truth from our in-laws, we have to make it safe for them to tell us the truth. We do not change in-law relationships by trying to control our in-law's behavior but by changing ourselves in relationship to them.

To listen to an in-law responsively, we must have what Mike Nichols terms *accurate empathy*. Secrets and distancing keep a new in-law from knowing you or your family, and it becomes next to impossible for the new in-law to have accurate empathy upon entrance into a family if secrets are kept and distances are maintained.

If family members are too hush-hush about family issues, new members are discouraged from saying much about themselves. This is certainly understandable. There are few situations where newcomers can feel totally relaxed and comfortable expressing themselves. Past experience teaches that it is best to keep ideas to ourselves until we have assessed the law of the land.

However, as a new in-law enters the family, it is important for the newcomer, as well as the family, to be willing to take risks and trust that this new in-law will be able to handle a variety of family issues and problems, recognizing that some of the problems are universal to all families. Repressing and not talking about certain issues takes energy. Listening to and communicating with in-laws takes effort. It is hard to listen without interjecting or bringing in our own opinions.

Sometimes a listening ear is all that is necessary.

Respect your in-laws' right to be themselves and your right to be yourself. The best in-law listeners are people who are responsive but are able to tone down their own message, and who do not feel a need to give advice or to be reactive. If you listen to your in-laws with tolerance and understanding, without trying to apply quick fixes, the in-laws might find that there is really nothing to change, and that a listening ear is all that is necessary.

If you want your in-laws to be true and open with you, make it safe for them to tell you how they are feeling. If you act too shocked or hurt or upset when they tell you how they feel about a situation, you will close the door to a more open dialogue with them in the future.

Please Translate What Your Mom Just Said to Me

One way of learning how to communicate with in-laws is to look at the kind of communication they have with other individuals. Communication with a spouse, if in-laws are married, may be particularly insightful. If your in-laws do not express their opinions or desires to those closest to them, there is no reason to believe they will express them to you. If they argue with the people closest to them, chances are they will argue with you also.

In *The Intimate Enemy: How to Fight Fair in Love and Marriage*, George R. Bosh and Peter Wyden make a case for the importance of fighting in a marriage. This perspective might be enlarged to include the pros and cons of fighting in an in-law relationship. Bosh and Wyden feel that, in order to be intimate, couples need to be willing to fight over issues. *Fighting* may be too strong a word for in-law relationships; many in-laws engage only in heated discussions. Hostilities and aggressive feelings within a marriage may be deflected from a spouse to an in-law if these are not dealt with and discussed. Being able to discuss loaded issues can be a sign that a relationship is becoming stronger.

Few of us are mind readers. In their study of 50 *normally happy couples*, Bosh and Wyden found that almost none of the partners had any idea what was going on in the mind of their spouse when the spouse was angry. They relied on game playing, fake fronts, and ritualized routines to avoid conflict. If this is how couples in intimate relationships deal with conflict, trying to bring issues to the forefront with in-laws will be tricky but not impossible.

Few of us are mind readers.

Laziness is another reason for deficient in-law communication. Communicating with in-laws takes time and energy, and we can always use an excuse like, "I don't see my in-laws very often, so why should I have to deal with them?" When these patterns are maintained year after year, unless there is a crisis, the energy needed to try to change or improve in-law relationships is not generated.

Some in-laws, like Natalie, make an effort with excellent results. During the early years of her marriage, Natalie felt her mother-in-law was too controlling, and some of it was done through food. "She decided what we would eat, when we would eat, and where we would eat," said Natalie. "One day, I just asked her if she could stop chopping onions for spaghetti sauce and talk to me. I told her, 'Mom, you know I think you are a great cook, but we really don't need such elaborate meals with everything made from scratch. We would be glad to get cold cuts for sandwiches and also bring some things from home to help out. We would rather spend time with you than have you always shopping and preparing for meals.'" To her surprise, rather than being offended, Natalie's mother-in-law was delighted.

Communicating with In-Laws by Mail

Things may be said in a letter that would never be said in person.

Telephone and letter communication can be used to further in-law bonding or can create mischief among in-laws. Things might be said to an in-law in a letter that would never be said in person. Some in-laws write letters in a stream of consciousness and do not have the good sense to censor some of their comments. Letters can be reread and passed on to other family members, and thus are open to a constant barrage of misinterpretation. Such was the case with the following sister-in-law.

Hanson said his sister-in-law drove him crazy. "She takes the most intimate information and then writes a letter telling that my brother-in-law [her husband] has hemorrhoids." The sister-in-law apparently photocopied her letters and mailed them to a variety of family members with a short handwritten note at the bottom: "Hi. Hope things are going well.

Here's the family news." Hanson did not confront her about it because he admits he enjoyed hearing all the dirty news about everyone else; however, he is sure there are other letters that go out with information about him or his family.

The best advice I heard about writing letters came from my father-in-law. He said when you write a letter to an in-law, put it in a drawer, save it for a few days, reread it, and then decide whether what you've written is what you really want to say.

I Heard It on the Grapevine—Over the Wire with In-Laws

One of the problems with communicating with in-laws by telephone, particularly long distance, is the time zone differences. The time at which you place the call may not be a convenient time for the in-law to speak to you. You may be calling at 8:00 P.M. from the Pacific Coast, and they are receiving your call at 11:00 P.M. on the East Coast.

Suggest to in-laws who are contacted frequently that a time be appointed that is best for all the in-laws concerned. One father-in-law called his son and daughter-in-law every Saturday morning at 10:00. The family enjoyed the calls and looked forward to the connection. However, it was agreed at the start that it was not mandatory for the family to be home to receive the telephone call or for the in-law making the call to feel obligated to make it every Saturday morning. When the father-in-law passed away, the calls were sorely missed and now are a fond remembrance of a pleasant in-law experience.

A time can be set up that is best for all the in-laws concerned.

Some in-laws have uncomfortable phone habits. Noland's wife Tess would thrust the phone into his hands and say, "Here, say something to my mother." The unwary in-law may be busy shining shoes or bathing the dog, but must put everything down at that moment in order to seem like a good and cooperative in-law. It is difficult to be sunny and cheery under such circumstances.

In-Law Relationships—Defining Moments

A personal contract can be lasting.

Ever consider that we all make unwritten contracts with ourselves regarding what kind of a relationship we will have with our in-laws? Often, these contracts are made at what I call *defining moments.* In a negative defining moment, my brother-in-law yelled at me and I contracted with myself that I would never put myself in that kind of situation with him again. A personal contract made during a defining moment can also be positive and lasting. A daughter-in-law, Bronwyn, told this story after 40 years of marriage. She recalled when her future mother-in-law visited her at college. It was close to Valentine's Day and the future mother-in-law brought lovely wrapped packages for both her own daughter and future daughter-in-law, Bronwyn. "When I opened the package, I found that my future mother-in-law had purchased a necklace for me that was exactly the same as the one she had purchased for her own daughter," said Bronwyn. "I felt that at this moment, she really accepted me as a part of the family and she would treat me as a daughter." The daughter-in-law made a contract with herself: "My mother-in-law is an OK person. I'm going to have a good relationship with her. We are going to get along."

In in-law relationships—or in any relationship—the defining moments and the comments we make about the relationship can be a turning point or a clarification of the relationship. On the negative side, a client said to her sister-in-law, "If you were not my sister-in-law, I would never see you again. We would not be friends." She did not remember the circumstances around this, but for her and for her sister-in-law, the defining moment said, "We are related strictly by marriage. We are not going to be friends."

These defining moments do set relationships.

Defining moments do set relationships. Think back. What are your defining in-law moments? What have you said or done that has defined your in-law relationship? Do you want to change those definitions? Would you like to redefine that relationship?

People make contracts with themselves for a variety of reasons. What one person thinks is a great in-law event may be a negative event for another person. In-law contracts are all very individual. If you want to rewrite your in-law contracts, you might want to start by thinking about and identifying your defining in-law moments. When did you decide that you were going to have a certain kind of relationship with an in-law, and what kind of contract did you make with yourself around that relationship? Identifying contracts and making them clearer in your own mind can give you permission to alter or change them.

Throw your obsolete, inappropriate, or outdated contracts out of your mind, and make a new contract of how you are going to *get along* with your in-law. If you are a seeing-is-believing kind of person, write down the contracts that you have now with each of your relatives. Then change or modify them, or even tear them up, and write new ones where necessary. These contracts need not be shown to anyone. They can be for your edification and can help you to clarify your feelings about each individual in-law. When you are identifying defining moments and clarifying unwritten contracts, remember that seeing people as a group—"the in-laws"—gives a faulty image. Let each in-law relationship stand on its own merits. Seeing in-laws as individuals creates a rich tapestry of relationships rather than a stagnant, sterile collage of "the in-laws en masse."

Make a new contract of how you are going to get along with your in-law.

Avoiding In-Law Splitting and Projection

It is not unusual for children-in-law or parents-in-law to be involved in what therapists term *splitting* or *projection*. In splitting, the person designates one member of the in-law couple as "the good guy," and one as "the bad guy." This is similar to the familiar good-cop/bad-cop pairing, but translates to good parent-in-law/bad parent-in-law, or good child-in-law, and so on. For example, "My father-in-law is a great buy, but my mother-in-law is a nag." Mothers-in-law are especially vulnerable.

Splitting is similar to the familiar good-cop/bad-cop framework.

When splitting occurs, the individuals involved should try to disentangle the personalities involved and identify a core problem area.

Projection is the attribution of characteristics (usually negative) to another person. Where there is negative projection, mothers-in-law are seen as the most problematic in-laws. Fathers-in-law are less often viewed as negative in-laws. In the older generation, economic issues may be a contributing factor. The father controls the financial resources, so any anger or discontent with the in-law relationship is projected onto the mother-in-law so as not to endanger a possible money source. Investing the mother-in-law with negative qualities may also be connected to the fact that women are just more involved with care of the grandchildren and with coordinating family activities—areas that can produce heavy in-law disagreement. Projection of anger or frustration onto the in-laws may also be a reflection of the relationship the child-in-law has with his or her own parents. In their psychotherapy work with in-laws, Linda Berg-Cross and Jacqueline Jackson have found that the tone of the relationship of the biological child with his of her parents will be a determining factor in the in-law relationship. This tone, it appears, often orbits around the mother and mother-in-law.

How do I recommend that you deal with splitting and projection? First, recognize when splitting and projection is going on. Second, ask yourself, "Am I the one who is doing it?" If you determine that some splitting or projection is going on in the family, analyze whether the criticism is justified and whether it has something to do with you. Are you not setting limits? Are you sitting by and complaining about others?

Often, along with the mother-in-law, the daughter-in-law and sister-in-law are seen as being bitchy and hostile. The fact that the female counterparts in the family are historically more active in the social roles may allow the males to lie low and not take an active hand in dealing with in-law relationships. Women can pay too high a price as the keepers of the kin, because they end up vocalizing the discontent and problems for both themselves and their husbands. In-laws, both male and female, need to speak for themselves and become involved in troublesome situations.

Some male in-laws stay out of emotional relationships that need changes. They withhold their opinion until the problem has become hopelessly escalated. When noninvolved males do state their case, they may take a dictatorial stance and recite a litany of *shoulds* and *oughts*, rather than coming in with a reasonable demeanor.

Learning to Give and Receive Criticism

Do you feel you are unreasonably criticized by your in-laws? Ask yourself, "What is it about the criticism that upsets me? What are my automatic thoughts? What is my automatic verbal response?" Many people, when criticized, think, "I must be a worthless person. If he criticizes my finger, my whole hand must be bad." These erroneous conclusions need to be corrected with a thought like, "That was really blown out of proportion. It didn't acknowledge any of the positive things in my life." As in-laws, we need to learn how to discover the kernels of wheat, then throw out the chaff.

In-laws need to learn how to decipher the kernels of wheat, then throw out the chaff.

Why do arguments abound when criticism is leveled at another? Whether the critic is correct or incorrect, a large percentage of in-law arguments would be prevented if the in-law being criticized did not get defensive. Bitter situations arise this way: An in-law makes a little criticism, and you defend; but now the in-law has to bash through your defenses. You decide to show that you can bash at world-class level, and before you know it, the conflict escalates. Most of us do not have PhDs in delivering criticism, so we need to be prepared to respond nondefensively to some poorly given criticism. Violet, a 21-year-old graduate student, said that one day, when her husband was being critical, her sister-in-law said, "I think my brother is out of line—just let it roll away like water rolls off a duck's back." The next time the sister-in-law heard him say something harsh, she gave a little "quack-quack." All three had a laugh, and Violet's husband knew the saying and realized he was out of line. In this situation, a little humor helped alleviate the tension.

Aggressive, Assertive, and Nonassertive In-Law Stances

Why are some in-laws so hostile and some so passive?

Why are some in-laws so hostile and some so passive? If you are a Harvey Milquetoast where your in-laws are concerned, assertiveness training can help you to deal with in-law problems. I did not say aggressiveness. I said assertiveness. That means getting your needs met while considering the feelings of others. Maybe you are reluctant to use a simple *no thank you* with your in-laws, and you feel guilty when you do say no. This reaction leads to passive-aggressive behaviors with anger generated, and sometimes results in blowups at unexpected moments. An assertiveness training course will help. Or, try reading books like *Be Your Best*, by Linda Adams and Elinor Lenz, which has many useful concepts.

Understanding the differences among aggressive, assertive, and nonassertive behavior, and finding out where you are on the continuum, will be helpful in all your relationships, not just those with your in-laws. This self-knowledge will give you an extra tool for staying out of in-law conflicts. Nonassertive people tend toward aggressive behaviors when they are finally pushed into action. Therefore, nonassertive behaviors can be quite risky for you and your in-laws, because when a nonassertive in-law blows up, he or she is bound to make comments or take actions that are not easily taken back.

Teasing

Some people fool themselves into thinking that their in-laws like to be teased. In truth, most people do not like to be teased but they will accommodate their in-laws by laughing and appearing to be good sports. Pamela's husband's family was very physical–huggy and kissy. Coming from a much more restrained family, Pamela was shocked at the first family gathering she attended, a picnic, when an uncle pinched her on the fanny. "To put it mildly, I was astounded," she said. "Throughout the day, six other family members—aunts, uncles, cousins, even his sister—also pinched my behind." In the back of her mind, Pamela thought, *What a bunch of perverts*, but they were otherwise friendly and nice. Afterward, Pamela asked her husband about it. He laughed, saying that it was just their way of being friendly and that they do it to everyone all the time. He said she should consider herself honored that they felt comfortable enough to include her in the family fun, and even encouraged her to do it to others. "They may find it amusing, but I have resigned myself to having my butt grabbed at his family gatherings, and secretly dread it," said Pamela.

The whole idea of teasing is based on finding a particularly vulnerable area and then using this area of sensitivity to bring attention to the in-law's Achilles' heel. On the other hand, certain subtle forms of teasing can be helpful, because they can let you poke fun at a family issue and loosen up the tension around this issue, thus bringing cohesion to the group. However, on the whole, teasing is destructive and causes anxiety and hard feelings within the in-law family.

Teasing is based on finding a particularly vulnerable area.

Can We Talk? Coping with In-law Communication Problems—Overview

In-laws are always communicating, whether physically or verbally, and the communications are not always in sync with each other. Dual messages between in-laws present the most problematic area in in-law communications. We communicate on more than just a verbal level; body language—our actions—can transmit a stronger message than the words we speak. Make a conscious decision on what you want to communicate to your in-laws, and then make your actions congruent with what you say and how you feel. Honesty is the best policy in nearly every case, but sometimes, as an in-law, you have to be diplomatic and recognize and reward effort and intention. Realize that some in-laws may need to be treated more like guests than intimate family members, and that more courtesy is needed in the in-law arena than in the family with whom you grew up. Recognizing and respecting in-law differences can dramatically change the dynamics of the in-law relationship.

Following are some questions to help you and your in-laws focus on how and what you communicate.

Worksheet

1. Am I willing to identify and work on changing unproductive communication patterns with in-laws?

2. Do I tend to split my in-laws by looking at one in-law as being good and another as being bad?

3. Do I project often unfounded negative characteristics onto an in-law?

4. Am I especially critical or negative toward an in-law?

5. Do I carry negative unwritten in-law contracts as a result of unpleasant defining moments?

6. Teasing—is it good, bad, or ugly?

7. Do I acknowledge and respect my in-law's style of communication? If I do not, do I work on making changes?

8. Have I recognized a need for improvement in my in-law listening skills?

10

The Holidays—An In-Law Adventure That Keeps on Going . . . and Going . . . and Going

Rituals for Our Times

The holidays are one of the times when extended families come together. If in-laws are geographically distant from one another, they may see each other only at occasions connected to the life cycle—weddings, births, deaths, or critical illnesses—or at holiday celebrations. Evan Imber-Black and Janine Roberts, in their book on rituals, distinguish between *outside calendar days*, holidays that are celebrated by the larger community, such as Thanksgiving, Christmas, Valentine's Day, Fourth of July, and Labor Day, and *inside calendar days*, more personal and unique family days such as birthdays and anniversaries.

Intense commercial pressure is put on families regarding the major holidays. Outside calendar days collect media hype, which generates high expectations for the in-laws and their families. With divorce and the formation of stepfamilies, children may have two separate households and four sets of grandparents and in-laws with whom they may be expected to interact. Adult in-laws may face complicated gift lists that include stepchildren and ex-in-laws.

Intense commercial pressure is put on families regarding the major holidays.

One way to ease the tension surrounding the holidays is to ask the in-laws, in advance, for help and direction in completing specific tasks or planning traditional activities. Borrow and prepare a special recipe, or schedule an in-law to share a song or conduct a game from his or her childhood. Including in-laws in planning can reassure them that they are important to the festivities.

Be optimistic regarding in-law relationships. Ask your in-laws what would make a holiday satisfying for them, and do what you can to make it happen. Be mindful of what you say to in-laws during the holidays. Every question you ask makes a statement.

Small changes can have a ripple effect.

Changes do not need to be big. Ask yourself, "What is the smallest change I could make to improve my relationship with my in-laws during the holidays?" Small changes can have a ripple effect. If changes occur, ask yourself, "How did that happen? What did I do or say that enabled me to have a different experience with my in-law?" Be willing to accept shades of gray with in-laws. If you argue, try to identify the arguments' constructive elements.

Watch for imbalanced ritual styles. Are you spending every Thanksgiving with your parents or your in-laws? Are you planning all of your family events for the children and not considering the parents-in-law generation? If so, is that what you, your family, and your in-laws prefer? Honoring preferences and taking suggestions from in-laws can give them a sense of ownership of the events.

Family Rituals

Differing expectations surrounding observance of rituals, including holidays and religious events, often batter congenial in-law relationships with friction and hard feelings. The chart on page 171 is a model for assessing which holidays or events are important to you, and for determining your expectations of how you and your in-laws will commemorate each occasion.

When you make your own list of holidays or events that your in-laws might attend, you may be surprised at the number of occasions

Holiday or Event	Important	Not Important	Expectation of In-Laws (examples)
New Year's Eve	———	———	Drink a toast at midnight. Hang up stockings for Santa to fill on his return to the North Pole.
Passover	———	———	Celebrate seder together.
Easter	———	———	Color Easter eggs in advance. Attend church. Have an egg hunt for the children.
Mother's Day	———	———	Treat mother or mother-in-law to dinner. Call if far away.
Father's Day	———	———	Exchange gifts with father or father-in-law.
Fourth of July	———	———	Cook out together, make ice cream, watch fireworks together at night.
Thanksgiving	———	———	Cook Thanksgiving dinner; follow the same menu each year. Go on a hunt for nuts and carolling after dinner.
Chanukah	———	———	Have dinner together. Exchange gifts.
Christmas	———	———	Select a Christmas tree together, have Christmas dinner together. Exchange gifts. Sing Christmas carols.
Kwanzaa	———	———	Celebrate ritual of candles, feasts, community celebrations.
Baby's Christening	———	———	Arrange for baby to wear family heirloom christening gown.
Adult Baptism	———	———	Invite cousins to sing a quartet.
Confirmation	———	———	Select sponsor for ceremony. Ask Grandpa to give a speech at party.
Birthdays	———	———	Buy gift. Attend all, unless far away.
Bar Mitzvah	———	———	Invite uncle to be toastmaster.
Bat Mitzvah	———	———	Invite aunt to help select caterer's menu.
Children's School Activities or Concerts	———	———	Attend some. Invite grandparents to major performances.
Graduations	———	———	Bring gift. Attend party.

Chart for Assessing and Planning Holiday or Special In-Law Commemorations when everyone participates. If the complete schedule is too strenuous, consider limiting the involvement of extended family to only a few selected holidays. One young woman was continually feeling shunned because the entire family did not attend all the special events in her daughter's life. She marked a calendar with the year's events and met with her parents-in-law to discuss the schedule. She then realized that, with all the commitments they already had, her expectations were unrealistic. She is content with knowing they will attend as many events as they can.

Only through exploring what you want, communicating your expectations to others, and receiving feedback on what those others consider important and meaningful will you have a chance to enjoy serene, conflict-free holiday occasions. At least you will have given it a try, even if some sweet moments turn sour.

Working with in-laws, in an in-law growth and development training program, Linda Berg-Cross and Jacqueline Jackson found that sensitivity to emotions stirred by holidays and special events can be important in developing mutual understanding with in-laws. In between special events, consider doing the corollary activities listed in the chart on page 173, or your own substitutes.

Do Not Fight Others' Battles

When you list your expectations, are they for you or for your spouse? Do you expect your in-laws to give gifts to and keep in touch with your spouse? Does it make you angry when they do not? Do not toss your in-laws out of *your* life because they slight your spouse on Christmas or birthdays. Let them fight their own battles. If your in-laws do not call your husband on his birthday, the omission is really their and their son's problem, not yours. Ask your spouse to look at the holiday and special events assessment you have compiled. Maybe what is (or was) important in your family is not a top priority in the in-law family.

	Important	Not Important	Expectations
Thank-yous	_____	_____	Notes are imperative for every gift, dinner; or, if we notes open gifts together, a verbal "thank you" is sufficient.
Phone calls	_____	_____	My in-laws will call with information on every new event in their family.
Flowers	_____	_____	I will send and receive flowers for all birthdays, Valentine's Day, Mother's Day, etc.
Photos	_____	_____	My in-laws will send me new formal portraits every year; therefore, I will always have double prints made of my photos to share with in-laws.
Letters	_____	_____	My in-law will write on a weekly (or monthly) basis.

Corollary Activities to Do between Special Events

Use the Holidays to Improve Relations with a Difficult In-Law

The winter holidays may be a good time to invoke the goodwill of the season and attempt to find some common ground where you can reconnect with alienated in-laws. It is often suggested that families adopt another family at Christmas. How about adopting one of your in-laws for a holiday event this year? Select an in-law with whom you have always had trouble—perhaps the one who has refused to come to family gatherings—or find a shirttail in-law whom you hardly know, and send an invitation to a family gathering. If you know that these in-laws abhor some of your family traditions, like the pumpkin-carving contest after

Thanksgiving dinner, consider giving up the practice or making a com-promise. A Thanksgiving or New Year's invitation with no strings at-tached has a better chance for a yes in these circumstances than an invitation to come for Christmas.

Try to connect with these in-laws in a quiet way. Make some small steps in their direction. This could be as simple as just identifying one thing you like or admire about them, or thinking a good thought about them every day. If you succeed with the holiday invitation, call the in-law occasionally afterward and say, "You have been on my mind and I just wanted to call and see how you are."

Make this an
in-law holiday.

I have proposed that you make this an in-law holiday by moving toward your in-laws. However, if you have tried unsuccessfully for years to con-nect with your in-laws, take this opportunity to analyze your relationship and perhaps change the ways you are trying to connect. Let this be the year you give your in-law a breather from the same obnoxious comments you have delivered every Christmas. When your sister-in-law walks in wearing the latest chunky boots, don't ask what days of the week she wears orthopedic support shoes to recuperate.

Because in-law problems are often exacerbated by alcohol, I recommend an alcohol-free or one-drink-minimum event. You can limit the drinking at your own parties by having a low-proof wine cooler or alcohol-free punch. Be sure to limit or deep-six the alcohol you may have elsewhere on the premises. Have plenty of alcohol-free eggnog, juices, cocoa, hot apple cider, or sodas available instead.

Notice the things that annoy or stress you during the holidays. If your kids get upset when your father-in-law does not call, call him first this year. Calling your in-laws first guarantees that they won't call you just as you sit down to Christmas dinner.

The holidays are not a good time to raise hot topics such as money issues or divorce. Stay with subjects that spread peace, joy, and goodwill to all, including in-laws.

Emotional Pulls

A number of emotional pulls are naturally built into the traditions observed during the holidays. Often, loyalty issues are involved. Among them are:

- **Pull toward the biological parents:** "I know my wife really feels guilty if we don't stay at my in-laws' house on Christmas Eve. But I am 35 years old and we have never spent Christmas in our own home or with my parents."

- **Traditional expectations:** "Christmas and Thanksgiving are for families. We have always been a close-knit family. I find it really hard to share the kids with their in-laws."

- **One big happy family:** "I'm not married to my son-in-law's mother. I'm sorry that she is a widow, but I just don't want to invite her to my Christmas party. She is a black hole of need."

- **Only one Thanksgiving:** "My husband's family expects us every Thanksgiving and so does mine. We just haven't been able to set limits. Can you believe it? We eat one meal at 1:00 P.M. at my family's house and then a second meal at my in-laws at 4:00 P.M."

- **Fair is fair:** "I know my wife hates the way my family watches television on Christmas, but I think she can put up with it every other year."

Lina, a speech therapist, has two children who are in their 20s. Recently, she found herself behaving like her own mother-in-law because she had not heard from her son and daughter-in-law for a month. "I didn't know if he had arranged their tickets to fly home for Thanksgiving, and I was getting very uncomfortable about not talking to him," she said. Lina was reluctant to contact the couple because her mother-in-law was "the travel agent of guilt trips. She constantly complained that we didn't spend all of our vacations and holidays with her, and I don't want to do the same thing with my children and their spouses." Lina had spent three years in therapy to avoid being as controlling as her mother-in-law.

After hearing this client's concerns, I told her not to overdistance, just because she saw her mother-in-law as being too involved in her life. It would not be helpful for her to detach herself from her children and not let her son know that she was looking forward to spending Thanksgiving together. Lina needs to find some middle ground between being too attached and too detached. She may tactfully give her son the message that letting her know whether they will be coming home for Thanksgiving is really a common courtesy.

Letting In-Laws Enrich the Holidays

Know about your spouse's holiday traditions if you want to avoid some common in-law problems. Think about or discuss these questions, keeping your partner in mind:

- What kinds of holidays does your family celebrate?

- Which are the most important or significant celebrations to your family?

- What are these events like and who usually attends?

- Which holidays are most important to you?

- How would you like to celebrate holidays? (Make it *wish heaven* and for a moment, do not consider anyone but yourself.)

- What do you think the high points of the holidays are? What are the low points?

Psychologist John Bradshaw calls these *celebrational rules*. These are unwritten rules and you should expect some early power struggles, however subtle, with in-laws over these ritual rules.

Family rules are often learned by just being around the in-laws for a few holidays and seeing what the different families do. What are your expectations about in-laws coming to your house versus going to other in-law houses? Who will shop for groceries, make the meals, do the cleanup? What courtesies are important? Is it important to write a Christmas letter to enclose in Christmas cards? What is usually contained in the Christmas letter? Do you sign the cards, or are they printed with your name? Do you save the ribbons and gift paper to reuse another time?

Family customs vary on how Christmas presents are opened. Does everybody gather and open them one at a time? Are they distributed wrapped and then all opened at the same time? Do you open one present on Christmas Eve? Do you eat breakfast together before you open the presents? What kind of presents do family members give each other? Does *everyone* exchange gifts? Do you give the sisters- and brothers-in-law gifts?

Do you not celebrate Christmas? Have you not had a tree because some family members celebrate Chanukah?

On Thanksgiving, do you watch the football games and eat dinner on TV trays rather than sit at the table, or is it important for your family to be seated at one table on Thanksgiving? Do you prepare special holiday foods such as breaded parsnips and sweet potatoes, homemade rolls, pickled cabbage? What are your favorite dishes? On Christmas Eve, do you have a big seafood dinner? Or traditional Mexican dishes? Do you go to midnight Mass? What makes Christmas *Christmas* for your family?

Now that you have considered your partner's holiday traditions, think of them in terms of your family.

- How do you approach your holiday celebrations? Whom do you need or want to include?

- How will you divide your time between your birth family and in-laws?

- Which traditions do you want to keep, change, or combine? Try to imagine your ideal holiday celebration.

- How can you communicate your holiday plans among your family and your in-laws? Do you believe hurt feelings can be avoided if expectations and changes in long-standing family traditions are discussed with in-laws well prior to the holiday season?

- Which traditions are you willing to compromise in order to keep the peace?

- Would you consider alternating the holiday coordination duties each year—your way one year, your in-laws' and spouse's way the next?

Use a Positive Reframe

During the next holiday season, you can use what therapists term a *positive reframe*. One client told me her son-in-law is from Argentina and never talks about family issues. Her daughter makes all of the decisions. I suggested that she do a positive reframe this holiday, by stating in a note her appreciation for how her strong and silent son-in-law is there for her daughter and grandchildren, and how she regards him as an important presence at family gatherings. It has been said that our greatest strengths are our greatest weaknesses. In a reframe, never, *never* say anything that is not true. Before I made my suggestion, the mother-in-law had told me that her son-in-law was very kind and available to his family.

Religious Differences

Religion can be a problem for in-laws during the holidays, especially if in-laws have differing religious beliefs. Chuck and Judy's troubles are a good example.

Judy was Mormon and Chuck was raised Catholic. Chuck always went to midnight Mass on Christmas Eve. Judy's family had a big dinner, opened a few gifts, and turned in fairly early. The first year they were married, the couple spent Christmas with her parents. The next year, they went to his parents.' "I didn't attend her Christmas program at church on Sunday, and she didn't go with me to midnight Mass," said Chuck. "After being married for a few years, we decided that this attitude was creating problems with our in-laws and that it wasn't important to take some kind of a religious stand. We now both attend religious services with whichever family we are visiting." For this couple, holidays did not seem like a time to work out religious differences.

Christmas can be a difficult time for Orthodox Jews, Jehovah's Witnesses, some Christian Scientists, and Asians and Muslims who do not celebrate the holiday. Take the in-laws' points of view into consideration when planning festivities.

Rita was from an Orthodox Jewish family. She married into a Reformed Jewish family who did not celebrate the Jewish holidays. When Rita got out a Menorah and showed an interest in celebrating the Jewish holidays, her in-laws became angry. They declared that they were Jewish by heritage, exclusive of practicing the Jewish religion. This issue had silently festered in the family, and now it flared again as Rita went ahead and celebrated the holidays. Rita's mother-in-law had a particular problem. She had somewhat resistantly given up celebrating the Jewish holidays in deference to her husband, who was adamant that they were Jewish in heritage only and were not practicing Jews.

After several years of marriage, the in-laws realized that their daughter-in-law was not going to give in on celebrating the Jewish holidays. But neither did she expect her in-laws to celebrate Passover or other holidays themselves. She simply invited them to join in celebration with her and their son.

When the family came in for therapy, we discussed what was really bothering the in-laws. The father-in-law feared that his wife would again want to celebrate the Jewish holidays and would bring up the same old issues. As it turned out, the mother-in-law was very happy *not* to celebrate

Mother-in-law was very happy not to celebrate the holidays.

the holidays. She had given up that custom years before. It was a burden to her at this time in her life, and, having raised her children, the observance was no longer important to her. When the father-in-law realized that no revisiting of old issues was on the horizon, he became more relaxed, compassionate, and understanding toward Rita's desire to celebrate the high holidays. In turn, Rita compromised at Christmastime by having a Christmas tree and celebrating Santa Claus's arrival with their little grandson.

Be Sensitive

The holidays can be difficult, depending on the year's events. If death or illness has struck one of your in-laws, this may be the year to suggest that you will prepare Christmas dinner. Or, let them know that you would be happy to fit your family's plans into their changed schedule this year. If you have suffered a setback or a loss, be sensitive to yourself. Maybe this is the year to spend Christmas away from home and memories, or to agree that adult in-laws will not exchange any gifts. If you cannot muster the will to recreate your old traditions, consider putting up a "Kitchen Closed" sign for the duration of the season. Let the in-laws know as early as possible, so they can accept the idea and make alternate plans. You may be surprised to find your family relieved to relax and go out to a restaurant for Thanksgiving dinner.

Give each person the gift of unquestionable acceptance as a valued human being.

Holidays offer some wonderful moments to get to know and appreciate your in-laws. Wayne Dyer, in *No More Holiday Blues*, suggests that you re-experience the excitement of your childhood, remembering how much you as a child enjoyed every aspect of the holiday season. I have adapted some of Dyer's ideas to in-law relationships. This year, look at what makes your in-laws happy rather than clinging to your own traditions and routines. Dyer makes this gift-giving suggestion: Give each person the gift of unquestionable acceptance as a valued human being. Let each in-law know that his or her worth is not based on meeting your standards or obeying your rules. Live in the moment and be available to enjoy your in-laws during the holidays.

Diagnosing Your In-Law Holiday Travails

I suggest a four-point approach if your holidays with your in-laws are not working:

1. **Identify the in-law problem.** What is not working for you at the holidays? Are your in-laws drinking too much or acting out, or are you less tolerant of their usual behavior because of the demands of the season? It may help to first express your problem to a neutral person such as a friend or minister.

2. **Own your response to the in-law problem.** Your mother-in-law frowns when you ask her son to change the baby in the middle of Christmas dinner. If her reaction makes you angry, realize that you are in control of your own reactions. You can change your circumstances or your response, but it is difficult, if not impossible, to change another person.

3. **Look for workable solutions to in-law problems.** Finding solutions to in-law problems during the holidays may mean breaking with your traditions or your in-laws' traditions. Consider your in-laws' feelings when you make changes. If you want to spend Christmas at home rather than at your in-laws' house, invite them to your home. If you do not want them there for the whole day, invite them to come in the late afternoon or evening for a snack or light dinner. Be specific in your invitation so that no wrong assumptions are made.

4. **Act, do not react.** Make changes early, to avoid in-law problems. *Early* means many months prior to the holiday. If you are bound and determined never to spend another Thanksgiving with your father-in-law, take a calm, nonblaming, nondefensive approach to the issue.

If you are married, you and your spouse can determine who should approach the in-law. When you have the opportunity, simply state that you want him to know early that you and your family are planning to visit your sister for Thanksgiving next year, but you hope to get together for dinner with him the week before or the week after. Letting people know early is the key. Remember, *early* does not mean the week before or the holiday week itself, especially if you are in the midst of an in-law problem.

Making Plans with In-Laws

Planning an in-laws' visit during the winter holidays can be difficult. For starters, do you know whether your in-laws will enjoy doing the kinds of activities that your family has planned?

In this age of dual-career families, holidays represent too few precious hours that parents can spend with their children. Stan and his wife desperately wanted to be alone with their young daughters and son during the holidays. The in-laws kept insisting that they would come and "share in the season" with the young family, and Stan felt selfish. "We had a limited number of days off from work, and I didn't want to waste one of them with them sitting around discussing their disease of the week," he said.

There are different agendas for holidays. Some family members expect to have a weight gain of one or two pounds; others make a personal vow not to have to diet after the holidays. Paula told me that all her husband's family ever thought about was food. "Every holiday is planned around what they will cook and serve at these mob scenes they call parties," she lamented. Apparently, the in-laws were all overweight, had very bad diets, and had never heard of the phrase *low-calorie*. Paula stated, "If I have to go to their holiday buffets and eat their greasy casseroles one more time, I think I'd rather just skip the holidays altogether."

There are usually only a few weekends surrounding major holidays, and these days can become precious as in-laws try to fit in parties with friends and time with family. Age and interest gaps may impact the guest list and cause some hurt feelings: one in-law may be invited or accept an invitation to a dinner party while others are ignored. Orson, an architect, said his family thought they should be included in every aspect of Orson's holiday season. "We had to keep our entertaining secret from them, because they would be pissed off if they learned we had a party and didn't invite them," said Orson. "The problem is that there are so many of them, the entire bunch overwhelms our tiny apartment, and we can't just invite one or two."

Divorced in-law families present a challenge for parents of underage children at holiday time. Responsibility usually falls on them to make sure the children spend time with all the relatives. Analisa, a paralegal, said, "Between my parents, my present in-laws, and my ex-in-laws, my daughter feels pulled into a thousand pieces every holiday—they all want to spend it with her, yet they can't stand the sight of each other." Analisa ends up spending every holiday in a taxi, taking her daughter to the three houses for portions of the day. "My daughter gets strung out and overstimulated, and then I get to deal with the meltdown once we get home," she said. "I think that, next year, we'll just go to Florida."

Roles

Holidays can be a time of friction regarding traditional roles. With the women doing the cooking and shopping, baby-sitting, and other "girl things," as one father-in-law put it, the men spend their time in male bonding activities such as attending and watching sports events. Leann, a 27-year-old psychologist, experienced this last year. Shortly before she and her husband left to drive 1,000 miles to spend Thanksgiving with her in-laws, her father-in-law called to say that he had gotten some tickets to the '49ers football game. "I was excited, because I really enjoy the '49ers," said Leann. "Come to find out that my father-in-law had not gotten tickets for me or my two sisters-in-law, because he had arranged for the girls to go shopping while the men went to the football game."

Roll Up Yer Sleeves

It is sometimes difficult to get in-laws to pitch in for special-event activities. I suggest making a written list before the holidays and then asking everybody to choose the tasks they would like to contribute, so that all family members feel some sense of ownership of the holiday. Yvette's husband usually was extremely involved in the holidays, particularly Thanksgiving. One year, he asked Yvette, before the holidays began, if she would mind if he did not participate in the work. He was really tired from a very stressful business year, and wanted to relax during the holiday weekend. Yvette assigned some activities to all of the children and in-laws, noting, however, that with her husband sitting in the living room, watching a game or reading a newspaper, her son-in-law also began spending more time sitting in the living room—relaxing and not pitching in.

Making Conscious Choices

You may need to take a holiday break.

Are you with your in-laws during the holidays because it is your choice? If you really hate all the preparation, responsibility, and cleanup and you do not have the holiday spirit, it is time to make a change in your life. You may need to take a holiday break. In academia, it is accepted practice for professors to take a sabbatical—some extended time away from teaching and campus activities to recharge their intellectual batteries and restore their creative juices. In-laws can sometimes benefit from holiday sabbaticals away from the routines. Next year, rather than spending Thanksgiving with the in-laws, go to a friend's or take a weekend trip. Perhaps spend Christmas Eve at home with your immediate family rather than going to your in-laws'; or, come up with a compromise.

Coping with Holiday Stress

In *Unplug the Christmas Machine*, Jo Robinson and Jean Coppock Staheli suggest doing two things to reduce stress during the holidays: (1) concentrate more of your energy on the things you personally enjoy doing, and (2) involve more people in the preparations.

Give yourself and your in-laws permission to have some privacy and thought-collecting time. Otherwise, you might start feeling like a slave. Make a sign-up sheet and let the in-laws pitch in with the work on Thanksgiving, Christmas, and other special-event days.

Encourage your in-laws to prepare their favorite dish, but let them choose what they will contribute to the day. Some in-laws would rather be involved in cleanup after a meal than in its preparation. If the in-laws do not like to be in the middle of the fray, suggest that they visit the local store for that forgotten bunch of parsley or carton of whipping cream.

The holidays are not a good time to try to reform your in-laws. If your son-in-law is from a family where men are above household chores, and your daughter has bought into his way of life, face it. Everyone is aware of the situation. You do not need to keep pointing it out. Resign yourself to the fact that, indeed, life is not fair, and your in-laws may not do what you consider their fair share of the work during the holidays. People can be inconsiderate. If your sister-in-law lets her children eat pumpkin pie sitting on your living room sofa, buy dry snacks and a good spot remover, and try to maintain a sense of humor.

The holidays are not a good time to try to reform your in-laws.

Holiday Gripes

The question really is, "Do you really have that many gripes about your in-laws or do in-laws just make good conversation?" I was in the supermarket two days before Christmas, walking around the dairy products when I heard one woman say to another, "My sister-in-law just left town." The second woman said, "Wow, I hope you put a Christmas wreath around your halo." The woman said, "Yes. I'm just exhausted. I've been cooking and cleaning and taking care of my sister-in-law. She's been here for a week."

By the time I got to the produce department, the same lady was there and I said, "Pardon me for being nosey, but I'm writing a book on in-laws and was curious about your relationship with your sister-in-law." I was fully expecting to hear some horrendous story about her sister-in-law. Instead, she said, "We get along just fine. I work for an auction company and she's interested in auction items. She comes to see me about every three months. I do a lot of cooking and cleaning for her, but I'm a widow and I really enjoy her visits. The people at the auction house where I work get a big kick out of hearing all my stories about my sister-in-law, how I have to do the cooking and cleaning and taking care of her, but we really get along very well."

For this woman, the stories about her sister-in-law were a good way to connect in a rather humorous way with her fellow employees.

Gifts for In-Laws

Gift giving ranks alongside baby-sitting as a potential source of heavy friction between in-laws. What to give and how much to spend can become major issues. Theron said that, last Christmas, his wife's family all agreed to set spending limits on gifts for each other. He thought it was great until Christmas morning, when he realized that he and his wife were the only ones who had followed the guideline of $30 per person. "It turns out that all her brothers and sisters spent four times that much, and we felt pretty sheepish as they opened the slippers and games we had carefully selected for them, after opening the bread machines, telescope, and electric train they gave our family," said Theron.

Gift giving is fraught with problems and can cause discord within families. For example, during the holiday season a few years ago, a client was annoyed that she had to spend the same amount of money on her mother-in-law as she spent on her own mother. I asked her whether this was required by her husband and she said it was not; she herself felt a moral obligation to spend equal amounts on both women. She felt much closer to her mother and wanted to reflect this in her gift, but she couldn't afford two equally expensive gifts. She was angry because she had to compromise on her mother's gift, and resigned herself to giving a rayon scarf instead of the beautiful Hermés scarf that she knew her mother would love. She said she hated Christmas and birthdays, because she always had this dilemma over the gifts having to be equitable. I pointed out that loyalty issues were involved, and I suggested that perhaps she and her husband might agree to divide gift-giving responsibilities, with each handling his or her own family's gifts. She agreed that this might work and said they would give it a try.

One set of in-laws handled the gift-giving loyalty issues by giving each of their children and children-in-law a dollar for each year of life on birthdays; Christmas gifts were calculated in the same way. Although this approach worked for this family, not every family likes to give money. Some people consider it crass to give cash gifts.

One needs to understand a family's traditions in order for the gift-giving effort to result in an appreciated gift. Gift giving represents a very important ritual in today's society, and those who take it lightly often regret doing so. Like the Japanese, who have a long-standing tradition that the gift wrapping is every bit as important as the quality of the gift inside, each family has rules regarding gifts, and these rules can make or break the in-law relationship. It behooves you to discuss expectations, themes, and even requirements for thank-you notes. In lieu of a discussion with

Each family has rules regarding gifts.

the extended family, your spouse can often provide the cues needed to successfully navigate this turbulent area.

As circumstances change, gift-giving rituals may be in need of revamping. Gwen said that the gift-giving ritual in her in-laws' family was getting out of hand. Gwen and her husband were expected to reciprocate with ever-increasing levels of gifts and could not afford the escalating spiral. Then, two years ago, when they bought their first house, they explained that their budget was very tight, and, rather than buy gifts for the extended family, they would make homemade Christmas cards and poems. "My mother- and father-in-law were delighted with the idea, and said they had found it increasingly difficult to continue the giving on that level on their fixed income," said Gwen. "Now, we all look forward to sharing the cards, poems, and stories, and my mother-in-law has created a beautiful album for them that has become part of their holiday tradition."

Some in-laws are impossible to buy for: they have everything, or no gift pleases them. Flowers, fruit, candy, or gift certificates to a movie theater are always reliable choices for an in-law who has everything or wants nothing.

Here are some other ideas for unique gifts for hard-to-please in-laws or for those who are on a limited budget:

- A living Christmas card (or mother-in-law's birthday card or Mother's Day card). Make a videotape of your family doing holiday activities, such as picking out or trimming the tree. The tape can be as elaborate or simple as you desire. Or, take your viewers Christmas shopping with you, on video. Suggest that they open the tape on Christmas Eve.

- A newspaper or magazine subscription that coincides with their interests: *Popular Mechanics*, *Utne Reader*, *The Wall Street Journal*, *Parents Magazine*, *Yoga Journal*, or *Self*. My son-in-law gave me a subscription to *Vogue* one Christmas.

- An evening of baby-sitting.

- An invitation to lunch, or a play, or just a walk in the park. Invite your in-law's family to a Christmas activity, such as a Teddy Bear's Tea Party or a performance of *The Velveteen Rabbit*.

- Four hours of work around your in-law's yard or house. One brother-in-law gave his divorced sister-in-law the gift of pruning her citrus trees right after Christmas every year.

- A positive message to and about your in-law, or a note telling an in-law something that you like or admire about him or her.

- A telephone call to tell your in-law, "I am thinking of you."

- A favorite holiday remembrance. Ask your in-laws what they remember as being special about the holidays when they were children. Recreate one of those memories by baking and mailing something special. Or, if they live near you, make them their special dish.

- A special Christmas ornament or other item from an in-law's spouse's childhood. Let the in-law surprise the spouse with this gift on Christmas Eve.

- A surprise for your in-law's spouse. Conspire to baby-sit for a surprise weekend while your in-laws go backpacking or relax at a bed-and-breakfast inn.

- A positive story about your in-laws. Write it yourself and read it at the Christmas gathering.

- A special note in your Christmas card to tell your in-laws of your appreciation for their role in your life or your spouse's life.

Have a Post-Holiday Planning Meeting

Two years ago, Christmas was very chaotic in my home. We had several young grandchildren and a lot of adults in a small space. It went fairly well, but there were a few problems. My daughter, who is a social worker, discussed with me, while we were out walking one day, what was going on and how we could help to ameliorate the problem. She suggested that we get together with all the family members to discuss the holidays. I thought the family meeting was a good idea.

When I got back home, however, I realized that the situation was too intense to hold a family meeting at that time. I hit upon the idea of a post-Christmas/pre-Christmas family meeting. Prior to our annual summer get-together, I wrote notes to all the family members telling them that we were going to have a post-Christmas/pre-Christmas family meeting, and invited them to come. I welcomed their suggestions and comments, and called for their views on traditions and their ideas for changes in our Thanksgiving and Christmas family traditions.

At our Fourth of July gathering, we discussed the end-of-year holidays that were ahead. I brought the videotapes from the past Christmas and the pictures of our Christmases together through the years. We spent several hours talking about the families, the Christmases past, and what we would like Christmas to be in the future. One of the in-laws said that he would like to be in charge of Christmas stockings for everyone next year, which delighted all of us. We also took the opportunity to exchange names so that, in our fairly large family, each of us would give a gift only to the person whose name we had selected. We decided to make this a secret drawing, to keep the gift givers anonymous. We agreed on a $40 gift limit. One son-in-law/daughter couple told us that they were planning to spend the Christmas holidays diving in Cozumel. We were disappointed that they wouldn't be with us, but we appreciated knowing their plans in advance.

If you have a planning meeting, let the young children be involved. They will bring fresh ideas and a lot of fun to your meeting. Also, let people know you do not need to do everything together. If some want to go to *The Nutcracker* and others want to go to *A Christmas Carol*, be willing to do that in small groups. You might want to figure out how to divide responsibilities and make plans and schedules, even though the holidays and events will not happen for six months.

Ask people how they would imagine an ideal holiday, and work from there. The wonderful thing about being human is that we can be flexible and we can change. We do not have to stay in the same old ruts and patterns, doing the same Christmas, Thanksgiving, or Easter rituals that were appropriate when in-laws had young children but are no longer appropriate with their teenagers. Write down all the ideas and schedules, and tuck them away in a safe place until the beginning of the holidays. You might want to make copies of these ideas and mail them off to the key in-laws in early November, to remind them of the holiday planning meeting.

Ask people how they would imagine an ideal holiday.

Creating Your In-Law Holiday Adventure— Overview

For some of us, the sights, sounds, and smells that remind us of happy childhood holiday experiences become very meaningful as the years pass. Because they link us to some of the best times in our life, we don't want to give them up when we become adults, and we tend to take them with us into our new in-law relationships. We may be recreating the peak experiences of a secure and carefree childhood. Or, wistful about what our childhood lacked, we may be determined to create perfect holidays and happy events for our own children. Holidays revive strong feelings and we often invest too much significance in one season or one day, whether it is Christmas, Yom Kippur, Ramadan, or Chanukah.

Differences in holiday traditions can bring an unbelievable amount of angst to the in-law picture. You may not relish the cheeriness, drunkenness, or bluster of the festivities. Some in-laws proclaim the holidays a commercial trap—a contrived profit time for the greeting card industry. For those who find joy and delight in the annual celebrations, the *Bah*

Humbuggers can cause distress. The time crunch that seems to get in the way of Easter egg hunts, Halloween costume parties, or a niece's bat mitzvah can also bring out the beast in in-laws.

Don't expect your in-laws to want to celebrate holidays and religious rituals in the same way you do. When two families merge, agreement is rarely reached across the board. Be willing to negotiate, be flexible, and have some give and take about building new rituals and traditions around both families' rich heritage.

Here are some questions you might want to answer before the next holiday season with your in-laws.

Worksheet

1. Do I make promises to myself, or my in-laws, that I cannot keep?

2. Can I do little acts of kindness for difficult in-laws? (Small is beautiful. Doing too much for them might become a burden.)

3. Do I respect the privacy of in-laws?

4. Do I set up in-laws for failure? (If you know they will be late for Christmas dinner, do not take it personally. Have a buffet this year instead of a sit-down dinner, and expect nothing in return, not even a thank-you note.)

5. Can I give up counting the minutes and hours my children spend with their in-laws and comparing them with the time they spend with me?

6. How can I be flexible with traditions?

7. Do I remember that families sometimes desperately need to have intimate time together, when they can relax and bond? (Do not impose your presence during the holidays.)

---

et
d)

ies, do I figure it is their loss?
and sisters or uncles or
years.)

d Thanksgiving are only two
ath, go for a walk, work in a

children or parents will
s? (You have developed your
you. They will develop

hey are easy targets when
want to say no to holiday

a shared history with in-

e joy of giving? (You will be

11

Money, Love, and Other Scarce In-Law Resources

Most of us join into this legally binding contract with our eyes closed.

Of all the contracts we may enter into during a lifetime, the most significant is the marriage contract. Marriage has been defined as the joining together of two people in a legally binding and recognized contractual relationship. The partnership that is created by the marriage is far more complex, and impacts more on the parties involved, than any contractual relationship created in the business world. Nevertheless, most of us join into this legally binding contract with our eyes closed, oblivious to the host of potential problems that might have been avoided had they been addressed prior to saying "I do."

When a couple becomes romantically involved, they share a desire to be as pleasing to the other as possible, presenting to each other what Virginia Satir has termed the *pseudo-self*. When it appears that a romance may lead to a marriage, it is difficult to ask financial questions. Problems often develop because of misunderstandings on the part of one or the other of the marriage partners. For example, if the bride-to-be has been given the impression that the groom-to-be is a wealthy financier, when in fact he is a sales clerk who robs Peter to pay Paul each month, problems are guaranteed to ensue when the truth is discovered. If the groom-to-be believes his future in-laws will welcome him into their business despite his prison record, he may be unhappily surprised.

Allocating Scarce Resources

In-law resources are scarce throughout life. There is a limit to how much money, time, and energy we have, yet these are the resources that everyone wants to tap.

Thinking about resources in terms of time, money, and energy can help in-laws and families realize that these resources are scarce and must be allocated thoughtfully.

Indebtedness and Money Management

Indebtedness and problems relating to money are probably the single biggest cause of marital stress and, therefore, have an enormous impact on in-law relationships. Although traditionally not a topic for in-law get-togethers, problems in this area can doom even the most promising relationships. In an ideal world, prior to entering into a marriage, couples would frankly and truthfully discuss the indebtedness and assets of each party, and would then prepare a complete and accurate listing of their joint indebtedness and a workable schedule of payments. Unpleasant surprises for the partner and in-laws would then be eliminated as the two enter into their married life.

Problems in this area can doom even the most promising relationships.

Second marriages are liable to carry heavy prior obligations. Student loans and credit card debt can also bring unwelcome surprises. Newlyweds who unexpectedly find themselves saddled with a heavy debt load may justifiably feel betrayed and may need to go to the parents-in-law for support. Prior indebtedness can also impact the in-law relationship, especially if the parents-in-law are expected to help the newlyweds financially. Why should new parents-in-law be expected to pick up the tab for their new son-in-law's student loans?

As a parent-in-law, you might encourage your children-in-law to reach an agreement as to incurring new debts or new lines of credit during the marriage. Point out that, legally, both of the partners in a marriage are bound to pay the debts incurred during the marriage, so neither spouse should arbitrarily and unilaterally obligate the payment of debts without the prior concurrence of the other spouse. Forearmed is forewarned: Here is how one in-law got sucked into paying in-law debts. Jocelyn's divorced daughter and her two children were living with Jocelyn. When the neighbor's son, John, who was in his 40s, drove up in his red Porsche to visit the daughter, Jocelyn was pleased. She thought that John would make a great son-in-law. He had a good job as a building contractor, and he had been divorced for several years. John and Jocelyn's daughter dated and, after two months, went to Las Vegas for the weekend to get married. After the marriage, the newlyweds moved into Jocelyn's house. Jocelyn soon discovered that John had lost his contracting job. With autumn's arrival came John's credit card bills and the monthly car payments for the Porsche. "Since my daughter is an only child, I suppose that the money and the house will be going to her anyway," said Jocelyn. "Sometimes it really grates me the wrong way to think that I'm paying not only for John's Porsche but also his $10,000 in credit card bills."

Put It in Writing

Lack of agreement will set you and your in-laws up for major disputes.

After you or your in-laws have had an opportunity to examine and discuss your individual financial statements, it is wise to reach an agreement, preferably in writing, regarding the transfer of ownership of autos, homes, business interests, stocks, bonds, and other assets. Misunderstandings can arise regarding property owned by one or the other party prior to a marriage, especially if some of the items are gifts from parents-in-law to their biological child. If it is the intention of the present owner to maintain sole and exclusive ownership of an asset, that fact needs to be clearly understood and agreed to prior to the marriage. This is particularly true when significant resources of the owner are to be devoted to preservation or securing of the asset—for example, the husband's cherished custom '67 Mustang, which requires $700 a month in repairs and maintenance. Agreement in advance regarding all assets will decrease subsequent misunderstandings and strain. Conversely, lack of agreement will, in the ensuing years, set you and your in-laws up for major disputes tied into issues of loyalty, trust, and priorities.

Whose Money Is It, Anyway? Breaking In-Law Tradition

In the past, in our patriarchal society, men have often had control of the money. A generation ago, this is how the parents-in-law handled their money. Because more women are now working outside the home, and have their own credit line, finances are more often being jointly handled. Your parents-in-law may have handled their money and resources in the old father-knows-best manner, but, in the 1990s, you may need to establish new patterns whereby neither you nor your partner has an exclusive right to control and allocate family resources.

Many new marriages involve financial responsibility for the existing children of one or both of the parties. If this is the case, the couple needs to clearly reveal their existing obligations and reach an agreement as to how those obligations will be met. Care should be exercised to ensure that any obligations incurred are not binding on the individual partners in the event of dissolution of the marriage and remarriage of one of the partners. It would be uncomfortable and unfair to be obligated to rear and support a child who is not one's biological offspring.

These questions arise: "Who pays for my child's tuition?" "What about tax liens from a bankrupt company I previously owned?" "How do we handle support of my mother-in-law in the nursing home?" "Do I have to contribute my earnings to meet my husband's child support payments?" Early and detailed discussion can prevent many problems.

When Chauncy got married, his father-in-law insisted that Chauncy borrow a dollar from him. Although it seemed unusual, Chauncy agreed. The father-in-law then said, "Now listen carefully. If anyone should ever ask you if they can borrow money from you, you can say, 'I'm sorry, but I owe my father-in-law money.'"

Business Is Business

When in-laws contemplate either lending or borrowing from other in-laws, or making investments in their in-laws' business ventures, it is of vital importance to everyone concerned that the transactions be in accordance with sound business principles. This means that every representation or agreement must be given a thorough *due diligence examination*—a complete investigation of all the business concerns before the agreement is executed. Although it may seem harsh, if you are considering investing with in-laws, employ the services of credit bureaus and business associations prior to the transaction.

Documentation eliminates many in-law problems before they arise.

"Do not take it personally. It is just business." Business dealings between in-laws are very dicey—it is easy to make assumptions that are totally off the mark. If you think business dealings with strangers may get you into hot water, dealings with in-laws are far riskier. If loans to or from in-laws are contemplated, wisdom dictates that there be a written agreement. An impartial third party should serve as a buffer. Some successful family transactions have resulted from reliance not only on a clearly drafted and executed contract, but also on the use of a bank or trust officer who transfers and receives funds on behalf of the principals. You may think the use of formal contracts appears cold and reflects a lack of trust, but, over the term of the transaction, the documentation and reliance on escrow or trust officers eliminates many in-law problems before they arise.

When Devon wanted to start a coffee house, she took out a second mortgage on her house and asked both her parents and her parents-in-law to invest in her business. After a somewhat successful first year, the business hit the skids and folded. Devon took on a temporary job to forestall foreclosure on her house when she couldn't make the business loan payments. She was unable to make good on her other loan obligations. In order to lend her the money, her parents-in-law had taken out a home improvement loan on their own house, and were now placed in a bind because Devon could not make the agreed-on payments. They expected their son to make good on the loan. When he was unable to, the parents-in-law became extremely bitter.

A Loan or an Investment?

A good question to ask yourself is: "Is it a loan or an investment?" According to my father-in-law, a cardinal rule regarding business dealings between in-laws is that unless one is willing to reduce the transaction to a legally binding contract that can be enforced, then one should consider the investment or loan as a *gift*, without any expectation of repayment or of realization of a return on an investment. My father-in-law's philosophy was that initially gifting the money saves a lot of hard feelings later. He liked to recount Benjamin Franklin's adage, "It is better to give than to lend, and it usually costs about the same."

It is better to give than to lend, and it usually costs about the same.

Paying for an In-Law's Education

If you or your in-laws agree to loan money or pay tuition for the in-laws' benefit, it is recommended that the terms of the agreement, as with any business agreement, be set in writing. Hard feelings can result when expectations are not met. Jethro, a very successful podiatrist, loaned $40,000 to his daughter-in-law, Kate, over the course of four years, to help pay for her college tuition. Not only did Kate disappoint Jethro by not going into the career that he had suggested, but she never graduated from college. Instead, Kate changed from one major to another. As Jethro and Nancy viewed it, she "played at going to school" at their financial expense and their son's emotional expense. Although Kate had

Hard feelings can result when expectations are not met.

agreed that she would pay the money back, no date of payment or interest rate was agreed on. Five years after Kate dropped out of school and took a job as an insurance agent, Jethro had a massive heart attack and was required to go on disability. At that point, Jethro and Nancy were extremely angry at Kate because the money that had been loaned was now greatly needed. An ever-widening rift that began with the good intentions of the father-in-law had expanded to a point where it engulfed the relationship. Kate now avoids any encounters with her in-laws and discourages her husband from dealing with them as well.

Professional Student? Reluctant Student?

When children-in-law have not completed their college degrees, parents-in-law may be called on or may desire to provide financial assistance in the hopes that education will impact the in-law's earning potential in a positive direction. This is not always the case and can be a frustration. Your desire to have your in-laws or potential in-laws go to school may not always be welcome. It may be seen as a message from the parents-in-law that the children-in-law are not up to par.

Keeping the Marriage Together

Giving or loaning money is not always negative. Sometimes, having the parents-in-law infuse some money into the couple's family can help to keep the marriage together. Carl's son-in-law, Gary, was a farmer. Carl's daughter hated the dusty, isolated, and windy farm. She felt that she had made a good try but just couldn't take it any more. After two years, she called home and said she was leaving the farm and moving back to the city and that Gary could choose to go with her or stay on the farm. Gary asked Carl what he should do. Gary was a farmer, and he didn't feel he could make a living in the city. "Since we had two grandchildren and our daughter to think about, we offered to send him back to school," said Carl. "We got him in as an apprentice in the electricians' union, and four years later he became an electrician and is doing well." It was a financial sacrifice for Carl and his wife to send Gary to school; however, they think it has been well worth the investment.

Money Talks, but Does Not Talk Back

Contractual, legal, and financial matters are important underlying issues for families. An an in-law, you can be unwittingly drawn into in-law control conflicts connected with financial resources, family businesses, and the time and resource demands that test the nerves of the most well-adjusted in-laws.

You can be unwittingly drawn into in-law control conflicts.

Pride and loyalty issues that involve financial support, or being helped out in ways that one's biological parents cannot afford, put stress on the in-law structure. Financially well-off in-laws who are generous with their resources often receive more attention, and the less wealthy in-laws may be distanced from their biological child. It is difficult for anyone to turn down weekend trips or paid vacations.

Prenuptial Agreements and In-Laws

Florence Kaslow, Director of the Florida Couples and Family Institute, suggests that you or your in-laws may address (and often circumvent) many legal and financial problems by drawing up a prenuptial agreement. Most people who have been married more than once or have accumulated considerable assets insist on the execution of written prenuptial agreements. These agreements clearly document the understandings of the parties prior to the marriage and usually establish a positive agreement as to the division of assets in the event of the dissolution of the marriage. Normally, the parties to the agreement execute it after being advised by their respective legal counsel. Although these contracts clarify the positions and understandings of the husband and wife, they are not entirely foolproof.

Prenuptial agreements are not entirely foolproof.

You may find that your future spouse or in-law, especially entering a first marriage, regards even the consideration of such an agreement as indication of a lack of sincere love and trust, or sees it as introducing the specter of divorce long before the marriage vows are taken. Meredith and Andrew came to couples therapy because, although they were in love and wanted to marry, Meredith refused to even consider a prenuptial agreement, despite the fact that Andrew had amassed considerable wealth and had had three prior wives. Meredith said that creating such an agreement would be dooming the marriage to failure before it even had a chance. Andrew was adamant, refusing to marry without the agreement. Primarily, he sought to protect his estate for his children from his earlier marriages. More importantly, he wanted Meredith to understand not only the assets, but also the tremendous financial liabilities he had incurred in his many business dealings.

I worked with the couple to help them separate the issues of romance and love (and along with those, the goal of creating a marriage that meant *until death do us part*) from the financial and legal entanglements that the prenuptial agreement would clarify. After much consideration, Meredith assented to the agreement and the marriage took place. When I last inquired, the marriage was still going strong eight years later.

According to Florence Kaslow, legal prenuptial agreements are highly personal documents and can be viewed as charts of the couple's future together. These agreements can be creative and can build the marriage on a foundation of trust and honesty. However, if the parents-in-law try to instigate an agreement, their uninvited involvement can be divisive and delivers a message that they believe the marriage may not last.

Is a Premarital Background Investigation Warranted?

"You must be kidding—a background investigation?" Look at it this way: When a person applies for a position of responsibility or trust in governmental organizations, the candidate is required to successfully undergo a security background investigation. This requirement is designed to ensure that the candidate can be trusted with sensitive or important duties. The investigation discloses information about whether the person has a criminal record or has something in his or her past (or in that of a close relative) that would remove him or her from consideration as a candidate. Few future in-laws are likely to entertain the thought of an investigation of a prospective in-law, even though people today commonly relocate a number of times and at great distances and therefore may not be known to anyone in the community for any length of time. If this is the case with a prospective marital partner, many of the same types of questions should be asked—and answered—prior to the marriage. (A checklist at the end of this chapter gives a good starting point for a very enlightening discussion.)

You must be kidding—a background investigation?

You might think that encouraging your family member to ask these questions of your future in-law seems overly suspicious or even ludicrous. The questioning may have to be subtle, because people on the receiving end of the questions might feel that they are being cross-examined. However, those who have nothing to hide will understand the need for disclosure of personal information and will usually answer with forthrightness and candor. Any discussions of this type should, of course, be reciprocal.

"If I'd Only Known"

One of my clients, Alyssa, wishes she had asked personal background questions prior to marrying Stuart. Swept away in the romance of marrying a man she had met on an Internet dating service for people over 40, Alyssa fell in love and married. Stuart, unbeknownst to her, had served two jail sentences and had left a string of wives across the country, some of whom he hadn't bothered to divorce. After the marriage was annulled, Alyssa determined that any subsequent marriage would take place only after a thorough investigation into the background of her spouse.

In-Law Insurance Issues

Discussion of in-laws' and potential spouses' financial statements should indicate the existence or absence of insurance policies and the coverage they provide. Couples are encouraged to discuss this matter with frankness and candor, because parents-in-law may be required to give support in the event of a death. If beneficiaries other than the spouse are to remain covered by the insurance policies, it should be only with the agreement of both parties, if earnings of the couple are to be used to pay the insurance premiums. If existing beneficiaries of insurance policies are to be changed in order to provide for the bride-to-be or husband-to-be, the couple should reach a clear agreement on this protection. The amount of coverage involved in insurance policies should also be clearly understood and agreed to. A husband's or wife's discovery that community income has been devoted to pay for insurance for the benefit of someone other than themselves can cause severe strain on marital relationships.

Kent was extremely devoted to his widowed mother. Before his marriage 22 years earlier, Kent had designated her as the beneficiary of his substantial life insurance policy. When his mother died in a car accident, Kent realized that he needed to change his beneficiary designation. His wife, Julianne, was shocked and enraged to find that she had contributed for so many years to ensure her mother-in-law's financial comfort. If Kent had died, Julianne and her daughter would have had no insurance benefits. Julianne justifiably felt betrayed.

Using Wills and Estate Planning to Avoid Future In-Law Conflicts

Under early English law, in-law relationships were significant. The father-in-law had jurisdiction regarding the welfare of a daughter-in-law and, in some cases, a son-in-law. The oldest brother (in most families, the property holder) also had some clout as to the welfare of the brothers-

and sisters-in-law. Today, the sense of being an in-law is usually viewed as an informal affiliation, not a formal legal connection. However, many financial and legal considerations must be addressed if one is to avoid the potential hazards that can be created by assumptions and misunderstandings.

Problems may surround family businesses or issues of in-laws being involved in wills and estates. Is there a will? Who is the executor? Who gets what, and when do they get it? Who gets mother's diamond ring and dad's watch? Who gets the family car and the antique rocker? These are only *things* and they are not worth bad family feelings. In-laws often get caught in the fray when they simply try to support their spouses.

These are only things, and they are not worth bad family feelings.

Chad's mother-in-law was a frugal person who had few possessions. In her will, in addition to her household goods, she left each of her children a small item. Chad's wife, Mary, received two small Wedgwood plates her mother had inherited from her own grandmother. Content with her Wedgwood plates, Mary decided she would give her nieces and nephews the option to take her share of the furniture and other household items that were left. However, Mary's aunt announced that the Wedgwood plates really belonged to her, because they had been her mother's. Mary told her that, because they were the only things she had inherited from her mother, she wanted to keep the plates. Every time Mary saw any cousins, they would bring up the fact that her aunt still wanted the plates. The conflict got to the point where Chad no longer wanted to have a relationship with any of his in-laws. Several months later, Mary decided on her own that it would be a good idea to send the plates to her aunt and end the whole scenario. "You'd think she'd get a thank-you from my aunt-in-law," said Chad. "Rather than that, Mary got a letter stating that they would not have had these problems if my wife had done the right thing in the first place. I can imagine how it must be for people who are involved with huge estates. These plates were probably worth about $400 and yet were able to create a ridiculous amount of in-law problems."

The story would not surprise any therapists who see in-laws fighting over some of the most ridiculous things. The things seem to be symbolic of the larger issue of sentimentality and connection with people who have passed on. A friend of mine who is a divorce mediator once told me, "It is not the big things that are a problem. The couples who are divorcing, selling houses, and dividing up retirement funds often find themselves fighting over who gets the hair dryer and the Dustbuster."

In-laws are sometimes called on to settle the estates of a newlywed couple who died without making a will.

Without undue delay after a marriage, the addition of a child, or joint purchase of property, a couple should make provision for the orderly transfer of their estates in the unhappy event of the demise of one or both of them. The euphoria that follows a marriage, the birth of a child, or a decision to commit to a relationship can lead the couple to delay or overlook the necessity of providing for the orderly settlement of their estates. It is generally advisable to seek the counsel of an attorney to assist in the drafting of wills. Family members, including in-laws, are sometimes called on to settle the estates of a newlywed couple who died without making a will. A surviving spouse or family member should have the benefit of a clear expression of the wishes of the deceased.

One client, Chester, an attorney called it "the dead hand from the grave." I call it just plain mean. Chester said, "When my mother-in-law died 22 years ago, my father-in-law could not deal with being alone and, after only six months, remarried a widow whom he had known for years. To protect their children's inheritance and avoid taxes, the couple signed a prenuptial agreement. My new stepmother-in-law left her assets to her children upon her death. My father-in-law left his more substantial assets in trust, with a stipulation that the income would support his new wife, my stepmother-in-law, until her death. Three years after their marriage, my father-in-law died and the trust became active. My stepmother-in-law received the income from the trust for the next 19 years. She recently died at age 83 of Alzheimer's disease. My wife's sister, who had been initially opposed to such a sudden marriage but had been highly supportive of my stepmother-in-law and her family during the ensuing years, contacted the bank regarding the trust. She was informed that, two years after my father-in-law's death, my stepmother-in-law used her power of appointment to change the will. All of the money had been left to her three children. My wife and sister-in-law received nothing from their father's estate." Fortunately this story has a happy ending. Chester recently told me that the step-siblings had graciously signed over the assets to Chester's wife and her sister.

Stories like this give stepmothers-in-law a bad name. Appointments, as in this case, may be made so the children can avoid taxes, but the strategy can backfire. Power of appointment must be taken very seriously.

People Get Weird about Money—"I'm Spending My Kids' Inheritance"

In-laws can get very weird where money is concerned, especially as they get older. The children-in-law become worried that the parents-in-law will spend their inheritance. One of my wealthier clients told me he makes an effort to tell his children, whenever he takes a vacation, that he is spending the money he has earned through his own labors. He and his wife plan to enjoy their money, taking little trips while they are here. They do not worry about leaving an inheritance for their children.

I have worked with families where the in-laws married with the expectation that their spouse would receive an inheritance they may push the spouse to be active in the family business or to move into the family home in order to establish *squatter's rights*. This can be very upsetting if a parent-in-law's spouse dies and the surviving parent-in-law decides to remarry.

Gladys really thought she was home free. Her father-in-law was 91 years old and seemed to be doing really well. Gladys was surprised and upset when he started to date a 40-year-old woman. Gladys had made plans for her father-in-law's large estate. She planned on private schools and an Ivy League college for her daughter. Now that the old man was thinking of remarrying, she wasn't sure where they stood. It seemed unfair; he had been a widower for the past 20 years, and she had been involved in taking care of him. Her father-in-law did marry the young woman, and one year later he died of a heart attack. To everyone's amazement, her father-in-law, a prominent businessman, had not left a will. Gladys's young mother-in-law now has the case in court and is arguing for a large part of the estate. Gladys realizes that a hefty share of the estate will end up going to the lawyers.

Incapacitated In-Laws

The stresses of life lie heavy on the husband, wife, or in-law who is confronted with handling the business affairs and providing for the care of a family member who is incapacitated by physical or mental disability, or who has become incarcerated. We have all talked about living wills—instructions that no heroic measures are to be taken to unnaturally extend the life of a terminally ill patient. However, most of us have not considered the advisability of creating legal documents that will empower each spouse or partner (or in-law) to manage the other's affairs in the event of incapacitation. These documents can provide for the receipt and transfer of assets and can cover wishes regarding medical or other care. They can ensure the orderly management of the invalid in-law's well-being. Robert Lynn explains some options an attorney might suggest: appointment of a conservator or conservators in the event of incapacitation, and agreements that designate durable power of attorney. These, together with living wills, can reflect the wishes of an incapacitated in-law to avoid prolonged medical treatment or extraordinary efforts to sustain life beyond his or her wishes, and similar considerations.

In-Laws and Guardianship of Children

As an in-law, you will want family members with children to make provision for the guardianship of those children in the event of the parents' death or incapacitation. Harry Krause warns that, in the absence of such provision, the decision regarding the guardianship of offspring is left to a court, and a court's decision often will not be in accord with the wishes of the incapacitated or deceased parents. An attorney can assist a couple in drafting and executing appropriate documents. The person who is named as a guardian must be willing and able to accept and perform full responsibility. Suitability of guardians should be assessed frequently; changes are warranted as circumstances change. This designation can save many in-law heartaches.

When Taffy's daughter and son-in-law, Lilly and Pepper, died in an airplane crash, leaving two young teenagers, Taffy, the grandmother, assumed that she would raise the children. However, at the beginning of their marriage, Lilly and Pepper had created a guardianship agreement that designated Pepper's brother and his wife as the childrens' guardians. Over years, Pepper's brother had added three children to his existing two, and he and his wife had divorced. Neither partner was ready or able to assume the care of Taffy's grandchildren. Taffy had to cross some very high legal hurdles in order to become designated the official guardian.

Yours, Mine, and Ours

A very tender situation arises in the establishment of a new family unit that must include children from a prior marriage. The situation relates to the rights and/or expectations of other dependents or relatives and in-laws of the spouses, as well as the rights of survivorship between existing children and children born into a new family. In stepfamilies, equal treatment is fraught with emotions and problems. Stepfamily support groups or professional counsel are helpful in dealing with these problems, according to Emily and John Visher.

In stepfamilies, equal treatment is fraught with emotions and problems.

Vince married Simone; both have children from previous marriages. Vince and Simone brought solely owned assets into their marriage, and they anticipated creating additional assets. Vince had been caring for and supporting a handicapped ex-sister-in-law who owns assets controlled by Vince. Simone had been the sole provider of an elderly family friend. Vince's older offspring were resentful of the prospect of possibly sharing Vince's estate with children born of the new union. Simone's offspring harbored the same misgivings. Both Vince and Simone wished to provide for their current offspring, as well as children born of their new union, and both desired to continue providing for their extended family members and to ensure that these provisions would continue after their demise.

I suggested that Vince and Simone work together to reach a clear understanding as to their wishes and intentions regarding provision for their various offspring and continuation of their other responsibilities, and that those wishes and intentions should be made known to those who were impacted by them. In a large extended-family session that included Simone's friend, the existing offspring discussed their fears of being left out both psychically and financially when new children joined the family. The family members discussed how they fit into the family structure. This discussion enabled Simone's friend, who had been dependent on Simone, to see the burden she represented. After listening to the discussion, the friend realized that she should turn to her own family, rather than leaning on Simone. Simone and Vince decided to seek legal counsel to develop a workable estate plan that felt right to all involved. Solving these rights of survivorship helped to cement the new family and smooth the road for Simone and Vince to enlarge their family circle.

Scarce In-Law Resources—Overview

In matters of the heart, no checklist is going to save you or your in-law from a scheming partner. One associate even goes so far as to claim that people lose their minds when they fall in love; otherwise, most people would never marry. Rationally, it is much more convenient to live a single life, without all the trappings that marriage brings. Plus, the glow of love has been proven to give us all rose-colored glasses so that we invest our partner with qualities that may or may not be present.

We all know that financial disagreements are one of the biggest causes of marital dissension and in-law friction. They may be avoidable if the partners are secure enough to draft and process a prenuptial agreement. If you are a parent of a near-future bride-to-be or groom-to-be, should you encourage your child to ask the intended partner about writing up a prenuptial agreement? I believe you should. I believe the couple's relationship is more secure, given this evidence of sharing and trust. The information gathered and the answers given from both signers must be honest. Marriage is a legal contract as well as a romantic involvement for life. Its best foundation is truthfulness between the partners. In the frothy preliminaries to a wedding, the prenuptial can be a sobering reminder of the commitment each partner is making to a new life together that may have to include some forgiveness for a partner's past.

The following checklist has been designed to help you probe some potential problem areas. If the future in-law is not well-known to the family, have the following questions been asked and answered by the couple, at least to each other if not in writing, as part of a prenuptial agreement?

Worksheet

YES   NO

____   ____   Have you ever been arrested?

____   ____   Have you ever had a DUI (Driving Under the Influence) charge against you?

____   ____   Have you been in the military? Were you honorably discharged?

____   ____   Have you been married before?

____   ____   Do you have any children?

____   ____   Have you had a number of intimate sex partners?

(continued)

Worksheet
(Continued)

YES   NO

___ ___ If so, have you been tested for AIDS or other sexually transmitted diseases?

___ ___ Have you ever been outside of the country? What were you doing when you were abroad?

___ ___ Have you ever been fired from a job? Why?

___ ___ Can I speak with a long-time contact who has known you all your life?

___ ___ Can I meet your family?

___ ___ What kind (and amount) of debts and/or assets have you accrued?

___ ___ Have expectations regarding finances and assets been discussed? Have you prepared a financial statement?

___ ___ Has agreement been reached regarding pre-existing indebtedness?

___ ___ Have you ever filed for bankruptcy? If so, what type?

___ ___ Have insurance issues been addressed?

___ ___ Do the in-laws have adequate estate planning, including wills, living trusts, or appointments of conservatorship?

___ ___ Has guardianship of the children been resolved? Are in-laws aware of who has been designated, and has approval been received?

___ ___ If money has been borrowed or loaned to in-laws or other family members, is there a written agreement with a repayment schedule and remedies if expectations are not met?

___ ___ Are there unresolved stepfamily issues?

12

When In-Laws Hurt the One You Love

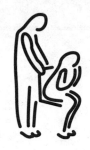

In-law abuse ranges from cruel remarks and subtle psychological abuse to physical abuse, sexual abuse, or alcohol/chemical dependency. Abuse knows no age or gender boundaries, and abusers take many forms, from seemingly kindly grandparents to jovial brothers-in-law or witty sisters-in-law. Questions arise that are often difficult to answer: "Is my in-law being abused?" "Where did those bruises come from?" "Why doesn't my daughter want to be alone with my brother-in-law any more?" "Did my father-in-law really drink two six-packs while he watched the game?" "Why do I feel so invalidated every time I see my sister-in-law?" "Should I butt in or keep my mouth shut?" This chapter explores some of the many specters of in-law abuse and offers suggestions to help you deal with it, whether you or a loved one is the victim—or the perpetrator.

As an in-law, you should know something about the abuse cycle, especially if you feel that there is physical abuse going on in the family. In the typical cycle, the abuser's pressure builds up. He or she becomes more tense and increasingly critical, and says things like "You've undercooked the food," and, when it is cooked longer, "You've overcooked the food." The partner is never able to meet the often unstated expectations, and the abuser looks for any opportunity to get angry. The anger builds, then explodes, and abuse occurs. Afterward, abusers are very contrite. They apologize; they say they will never do it again. They bring gifts. And then the cycle starts all over again. The tension starts to build. The person becomes hypercritical . . . and the cycle continues.

Abuse knows no age or gender boundaries.

Sometimes, as they feel the tension build, abused persons will aggravate their abusers in order to expedite the vent of anger. When abusers finally blow and the tension is released, it is possible to live with them for a while. This is how it happens that some in-laws begin to feel that they have triggered the abuse, when that is not actually the case.

Physical Abuse

When there are difficulties in a marital relationship, the in-laws can become intricately involved. That was the case with Ted and Lucy. Ted was referred to therapy to help him deal with his anger toward Lucy, who had taken their twin girls and rejoined her family in Montana after Ted had shaken her and hit her in the face, giving her a black eye. Ted was angry at Lucy's parents; he said his in-laws had encouraged Lucy to leave him, which was true. He felt that the fact that he was a Native American prejudiced his father-in-law toward him. Lucy's parents saw this as a decoy to avoid dealing with the real issue of spousal abuse. Ted had made a visit to Montana in order to encourage his wife to return to him. At the time, the father-in-law stated, "I don't want you abusing my daughter." Ted, who was the product of a broken home and an abusive father, felt hurt by his father-in-law's comments and his unwillingness to talk the situation over. After all, there were grandchildren to consider, as well as Lucy. Because Ted had a history of abuse in his first marriage, Lucy, with her parents' support, divorced Ted and stayed in Montana.

In this situation, loyalty to their daughter seemed to cause these parents to encourage separation and divorce. However, they had to remember that their son-in-law, Ted, will always be the parent of their grandchildren and, as such, cannot be ignored. I encouraged Ted to see his in-laws' point of view. Ted felt that his father- or mother-in-law should not take sides in a martial disagreement. I pointed out that this is a loyalty issue linked to the natural affinity toward one's offspring. Ted dropped out of therapy. He said that he really did not need help and had only agreed to therapy as a way to get his family back by letting them know that he was working on his problems.

Many women in our society are hit once or twice and then leave the abusive relationships. Hence, therapists more often see people who are undergoing abuse but are unable, for various reasons, to leave the abusive relationship. If you have an in-law who is involved in recurring abuse, he or she definitely needs some kind of treatment. The person being abused and the abuser need to understand why they are staying in this kind of situation, and what some reasonable options might be.

As far as women abusing men, there are relatively few reported cases of men being battered by their wives or female partners. Generally, when these stories are tracked down, we learn that the women have been so harassed by men that they finally strike back, and then men use the retaliation as an excuse to beat up the wife or partner.

If an in-law is doing the battering, you need to confront him or her and say that it is not acceptable. Usually, someone in the family has the power to stop the battering. A mother or a father may have great influence over a person who is battering a spouse or partner.

You need to confront your in-laws and tell them that it is not acceptable.

A couple came into therapy because the husband was hitting the wife. I asked his parents to come into the therapy session, and suggested that if the son tried to hit his wife, she and the couple's children could go to her mother-in-law's house, where she could be protected from her husband. The mother-in-law was not pleased with the idea that her grandchildren would come and mess up her house, especially if she wasn't at home. She was unwilling to give her daughter-in-law a key to the house, so I suggested that they might take a blanket and sit out on the porch until the mother-in-law arrived home. The mother-in-law said that she would be embarrassed if the neighbors saw the children sitting on the porch. I then queried the mother-in-law and father-in-law as to what they wanted to do about the physical abuse. The mother-in-law turned to her son and said, "Why don't you just stop it?" From that beginning, the son did stop abusing his wife, and the family continued in couples treatment.

The husband also joined a support group for men who needed to overcome violence, and the wife attended several group meetings at the battered women's shelter.

Sexual Abuse

Sexual abuse can be overt or subtle.

Sexual abuse is against the law. Sexual abuse can be overt, such as molestation or rape, which are police matters, or it can be subtle, such as exposing oneself to a child or commenting lewdly on a teenager's body. If the victim is a minor or a dependent adult, such as an elderly or mentally retarded in-law, overt sexual abuse must be reported to child or adult protective services. It is mandated that therapists report sexual abuse.

In-laws who sexually abuse or have a history of sexual abuse should not be allowed to be alone with family members who are vulnerable, such as children and dependent adults, throughout the perpetrator's lifetime. A person who is known to have committed sexual abuse or is a convicted offender has lost the right to ever again be alone with a child or a dependent person.

In-laws need to think twice before they allow family members who are known to have been sexual offenders in the past to stay overnight at their home. They also need to question whether it is wise to leave dependent persons alone with an in-law who has been raised in a home where there has been sexual abuse. A few moments can change a person's life, so it is prudent to err on the side of caution.

I recently saw a 33-year-old man who entered therapy as a result of being molested by his older brother, who had been molested by his grandfather, who had also molested the boys' mother. The young man, my client, had in turn molested his brother's two daughters. My client had been married for four years, and the molestations had recently become disclosed and reported. The older brother had apparently sought treatment and had contacted his younger brother in order to discuss his regrets about having molested him. My client's wife knew that her husband had been molested prior to their marriage.

I discussed with the younger brother how he would feel if his wife were to tell the in-laws (her family) about the fact that he had been molested and was himself a molester. He said that his wife did not want to talk about it. She wanted to keep it a secret within their immediate family. I reminded him that not telling his in-laws about his history of molestation could be destructive because it could continue to foster shame and guilt. The fact that he had in turn molested his nieces, a criminal act, poses a difficult problem that negates a decision to not tell the in-laws. Because he was reported to authorities, he will no doubt be mandated into treatment. The process will be difficult for his wife if she is not able to share this information with her family, for it will perpetuate the shame and secrecy surrounding his acts of incest and sexual abuse.

A husband or wife who feels that an in-law has damaged his or her spouse has an especially difficult situation. Isabelle, a 42-year-old mother of four children, was molested throughout her childhood by her father. When she married James, he became a self-appointed *protector* against the other man in her life, his father-in-law. When Isabelle's father became ill, James refused to go with her to the hospital, and when his father-in-law died, James refused to go to the funeral. James felt that, by his absence, he was showing his father-in-law and the family that he did not condone his father-in-law's outrageous behavior.

Isabelle was devastated that James did not attend her father's funeral, and she did not agree with his protectionism theory. She felt that she had needed emotional support in order to deal with her father's illness and eventual death. The fact that James did not give her support during this time took a large toll on their relationship. James may have felt that he had made a statement by not attending these events; however, one might well question whether the price he paid in order to make this statement was too high.

Where there has been a history of abuse or there are painful memories of sexual indiscretion, unaware in-laws may walk into a situation not realizing that they are expected to play a role in a script that the parents or the parents-in-law have written for the child's relationship. In-laws' past histories can affect how they feel about dating, relationships, and the sexuality of their in-laws.

One family came to therapy because the mother-in-law could not tolerate any visible affection between her daughter, Annie, and her son-in-law, Rob. When Annie sat on Rob's lap in a playful way, the mother-in-law said, "I won't have this kind of overt sexuality going on in my home." In looking at the family history, we learned that, as a child, the mother-in-law went to her father's farm to pick apples. Her brother, as well as a 16-year-old hired girl, also went to the farm. While the son and daughter were in the orchard, the father was in the farmhouse having a sexual experience with the 16-year-old hired girl.

The client talked about how painful it was to make the one-hour trip to and from the farm several days a week in order to take care of the apple orchard. This woman considered any displays of sexuality or touching offensive; they brought back her memories of her 40-year-old father taking advantage of the 16-year-old girl. This mother-in-law was able to see that the problem was with her own unresolved family history issues, not with Rob and Annie.

If you have inappropriate responses to such things as physical touching or harmless sexual innuendos, you may want to get in touch with a therapist and talk about those responses, rather than compromise your relationship with your in-laws.

Emotional Abuse

Emotional abuse can leave deep unhealed wounds.

Emotional abuse among in-laws is much more subtle than physical abuse. Many of the women whom I worked with at a battered women's shelter in Rochester, New York, said that the emotional abuse they received was far worse than the physical abuse. We seldom hear of anyone dying from emotional abuse, but emotional abuse can leave deep unhealed wounds that cripple the psyche of an in-law. But what is considered emotional abuse by you may not be experienced as emotional abuse by another person. It is hard to know whether your in-laws are being emotionally abused, because emotional abuse is subtle and happens over time.

Stay alert to signs of abuse, but do not try to take away from your in-laws the power to discipline their own children in fair, nonphysical, and reasonable ways. If you discourage in-laws too much without encouraging them to parent, you may find that they feel incompetent and withdraw. From in-laws who have ideas and opinions, they change into passive and noninvolved people. Encourage the positive things that you see them do and discourage the negative actions. Help them to move into more competent and reasoned attitudes. If they acknowledge a need for guidance, suggest that you will baby-sit while they attend parenting classes.

What can one do if an in-law is using negative parenting skills? Olive noticed that her son-in-law seemed to enjoy scaring his four-year-old son about raccoons, foxes, skunks, and other small animals in their backyard. The boy became frightened about going outside at all. Then, one day when she was visiting, Olive went to the nursery, where there was a little door that opened to the outside. She heard her son-in-law tell the child that if there were a fire or an earthquake, he should run out the door in order to be safe. To Olive, it looked like a tender scene. The little boy was absolutely entwined in her son-in-law's arms and welded to him. Then she realized that her grandson was terrified.

People do try to warn their children or grandchildren of the dangers "out there" in the world. It *is* an unsafe world; however, scaring children into immobility is not the answer. Like the lion in *The Wizard of Oz,* we are capable of courage, but we have to find that courage within ourselves in order to stand against the uncertainties of this world. When children learn fear before they learn courage, they are left feeling immobilized, vulnerable, and invalidated. Children can learn to be aware of "stranger danger," but that can be taught along with skills of courage and self-determination.

Frightening or worrying people can make them dependent on us. Sometimes, in the short run, that dependency feels good. But in the long run, when a child enters kindergarten or nursery school and feels fearful, some of the fright instilled earlier in an effort to protect the child may come back to haunt. On the other hand, some children, I believe, are by nature shy or fearful, and not all of their fears are planted by comments, stories, or what they hear the in-laws say.

Financial abuse happens when one in-law has total control of the purse strings.

One aspect of emotional abuse might be called financial abuse. It happens when one in-law has total control of the purse strings and does not allow the partner to have any money or to understand his or her financial circumstances. The abusing in-law constantly worries that there is not enough money to support the family's needs, or is frightened about financial security.

One woman I saw was feeling so strapped for money that she began sneaking around, looking at her husband's checkbook and financial records when he was at work. Her husband, a dentist, was in practice with her father-in-law. She told me that she got so frustrated about their finances and about having to beg her husband for money every time she bought the kids a pair of shoes that she finally pulled her father-in-law aside at a family gathering and asked him if the business was doing well. When he said yes, he seemed somewhat puzzled. She explained to him that she had been concerned, because her husband had said they had no money to buy the children clothes for school or to do any family activities. The father-in-law said, "Why, of course, there is money. Our business is doing very well. Let me have a talk with Daniel about this problem."

When her father-in-law told her husband that he had been asked about the finances, the husband was angry with his wife because she had talked to his father. She told him that she could no longer live with the way things were. She needed to known more about the ongoing finances.

Her husband was adamant. This was his money and she had no call on it. Things went from bad to worse, and she ended up filing for divorce. She said her father-in-law came to her and let her know that he had tried to work with his son on sharing resources and information about the family finances, but he had been stonewalled.

About a year after the divorce, the husband was still so angry that he sold his house and left the state, in order to avoid paying his wife alimony and child support. In this way, he was continuing with his financial abuse. The father-in-law is now helping the family out and is hoping that his son will reemerge.

Child Neglect and Abuse

When are you justified in turning your in-laws in to child protective services for ongoing incidents that are reportable? If you start creating problems for your in-laws, that part of the family may detach itself, or the children involved may end up being taken out of the home. Use common sense in dealing with in-law problems. Call child protective services anonymously, explain the situation to them, and get their feedback. They may be able to recommend some parenting classes or actions that will support your in-laws and protect the minors in your family. Be aware that once child protective services are notified, they are obliged to respond to the situation. Children are sometimes removed from the home and sent into foster care, or parents, if suspected of abuse, can be arrested and held in jail.

A client, Rosie, said she had a problem. Her daughter-in-law, Sheila, and Rosie's son were divorced. Sheila had custody of the children and lived a thousand miles away. Rosie's grandchildren, ages six and seven, were going home from school to an empty house. Rosie encouraged Sheila to move closer to her, saying she would be glad to help her raise her children, but the ex-daughter-in-law said that she preferred living in another state. One day, Rosie took a vacation and visited Sheila and the grandchildren. When she arrived at the house at 2:00 in the afternoon, she knocked on the door and nobody answered. The door was unlocked, so Rosie went in and found her granddaughter and grandson on a bed, taking a nap while their mother was at work.

I told Rosie that this was reportable child neglect. It is illegal for parents to leave under-age children unattended. Her grandchildren did need to be under some type of supervision, and I suggested that Sheila should be told that anyone—a neighbor or a school teacher—might report the situation. She might then be in trouble with child protective services and might lose her children.

Rosie called Sheila from my office to tell her that if she did not get child care, she would report the case. She was informed by her ex-daughter-in-law that she had moved in with her boyfriend, who also had small children, and that she would be staying home to care for all the children. Rosie told Sheila she was glad that this happened because she had been concerned. When I last saw this client, she reported that she had recently gone to see her grandchildren. They seemed to be doing better and were much happier.

Child abuse seldom stops on its own.

I recommend that you call your local child welfare office if you think that child abuse is occurring. Child abuse seldom stops on its own. Even though a perpetrator may stop for a short period of time, there is still a threat to those living in the home. Once abuse has happened, it could happen again.

Abuse of Grandchildren and Other Dependents

You may not be able to avoid problems with your in-laws if some danger or abuse involves your children or a minor. The in-law may not be your concern, but a boyfriend or girlfriend may be the threat. Carla and her husband were headed off for a romantic weekend. They dropped their three boys off at Carla's mother-in-law's house. She had agreed to take care of them for the weekend. When the couple arrived at the house, they found that Carla's sister-in-law's new boyfriend was also staying at the house for the weekend. "We had never met the man and when we were introduced to him, he seemed cordial and friendly enough on the surface, but something about him made me very uncomfortable," said Carla. "My husband and I both had a shaky feeling about having a stranger we did not know staying at the house with our sons; however, we didn't want to create problems or make a fuss so we said our good-byes and headed off for the weekend." Only a block away, the couple felt uncomfortable about the situation and drove to a pay phone, called Carla's mother-in-law, and asked her what she knew about the sister-in-law's boyfriend. "We knew we risked offending my sister-in-law, but felt it was more important that our children were safe," said Carla. They asked the mother-in-law to have the children sleep downstairs in her bedroom, rather than in the guest room upstairs. She agreed and although the sister-in-law was very offended, it worked out. The mother-in-law took total responsibility for the boys over the weekend. "I hope my sister-in-law will forgive us for being suspicious of her boyfriend," said Carla, "but she also has to consider that my sons had top priority in that situation."

In-Laws Who Abuse Alcohol and Drugs

The perspective of an outsider—in this case, an in-law—can point out the changes that need to be made in the family.

A new in-law who comes into the family may be able to identify some common collusion that he or she may either become a part of or take a stand against. These collusions might include drinking with a problem drinker, or demanding or inappropriate behavior. When in-laws collude by participating in behavior that they otherwise find objectionable, they inhibit their own emotional growth and the growth of the in-law relationships. However, an in-law is in a bind if he or she approaches the collusion directly. This action may be seen as disloyal; yet, if the collusion continues, he or she may be compromising personal ideals and values.

In-laws are in a bind if they approach collusion directly.

A client said that her husband was an alcoholic. Every time he drank, he got verbally abusive, and when she got upset, he went to her mother-in-law's or sister-in-law's house. My client was an adult child of an alcoholic father, and could not tolerate her husband's verbal abuse. In her mind, the problem was her mother-in-law's and sister-in-law's relationship with her husband, rather than the fact that her husband had an alcohol problem. Viewing the situation as a problem involving her mother-in-law and sister-in-law was easier to deal with. There was somebody to get angry at.

The problem was her husband's addiction to alcohol.

After discussing the issue, she realized the problem was not her mother-in-law and sister-in-law. The problem was her husband's addiction to alcohol. She then concluded that it might be helpful to have her mother-in-law and sister-in-law on her side, working to plan an intervention with her husband. I gave her the name of an alcohol intervention specialist, and when I last talked to her, she and her mother-in-law and sister-in-law, without the husband's knowledge, were planning an intervention.

If you do not want to approach your in-law's drinking problem directly, you can at least limit his or her access to alcohol in your home. Horace told me that because he knew his brother-in-law had a drinking problem, the family avoided serving alcohol whenever he was a guest. For Horace, it was better to avoid the problem than to talk about it.

It is not unusual for extended family to be asked to support family members who have a history of substance abuse. This can be especially frustrating for hard-working in-laws who see this type of support as enabling continued abuse. Such was the case with the following family.

Todd made an appointment for himself and his wife, Candy, to discuss his anger at being asked to pitch in to support his alcoholic father-in-law and his mother-in-law. What really frosted Todd was that he hadn't been given a choice; Lex, Candy's older brother, *demanded* that they pitch in and help provide financial support. Todd said that his brother-in-law just did not get it; giving the father-in-law financial support was making him dependent and enabling him to continue drinking. Candy felt caught between her loyalty to her brother and parents, and her loyalty to

Todd. Both Todd and Candy saw Lex as overbearing, always running around telling everyone in the family what to do. Todd also saw his parents-in-law being made into infants by their dependency on his brother-in-law.

In-law loyalties and hierarchies played an important part in formulation of this case. Lex's loyalty to his parents kept him firmly bound as a family care taker. The age hierarchies had been switched. Lex had become the economic supporter of his parents, and he expected his sister and brother-in-law to share the obligation. Todd, as an in-law, brought a fresh point of view. He recognized that his father-in-law was an alcoholic and needed to be confronted. This illustrates how in-laws can bring in new information and the news of difference.

The age hierarchies had been switched.

I suggested to the couple that, at the next session, Lex and the parents-in-law should join us, to see whether we could begin to discuss the family's problems. Lex said that he would come, but he did not think it was appropriate to involve his parents.

During the session, Candy told Lex of her conflict of loyalty between her birth family and Todd. She said that she did not want her marriage to end in divorce, as had Lex's marriage. Candy further stated that she appreciated the sacrifices that Lex made for her parents, but she felt that the price he had paid for his loyalty was too high. Todd then talked about his concern and love for the father-in-law. If the family did not stop denying the alcoholism, he feared that his father-in-law would die of alcoholism.

Although at first defensive, Lex had to admit, after a discussion of the signs of alcoholism, that his father was an alcoholic. He further admitted that he was tired of trying to hold things together in the family. They all agreed that the father-in-law should stop drinking and get a steady job. I suggested that they contact an alcohol counselor and do an alcohol intervention, and I stayed in contact with the family. The first intervention was not successful because the father-in-law refused treatment. The family then upped the ante: Lex told his father that if he did not go in for treatment, he would encourage his mother to leave him and would financially support her but would cut off support of the father. When I last spoke to Todd, his father-in-law was in a 30-day residential treatment program.

When In-Laws Should—and Should Not—Butt In

There is no place for physical abuse in any relationship.

What should you do if you think an in-law is being abused? There is no place for physical abuse in any relationship, with an in-law or otherwise. If you feel that one of your in-laws is being abused physically, you need to step forward and let people know that you will not keep it a secret, that you will bring it up whenever you see any signs that it is happening, and that you will not put up with it by pretending to be unaware or by remaining silent.

If you think there may be physical abuse, watch for physical signs: bruising, swelling, or difficulty walking. Some in-laws tell people they fell down or hurt themselves, because they are too ashamed to say they were physically abused by their partner, child, or parent. When you see these signs repeatedly and suspect abuse, be courageous and follow through. Ask questions clearly and openly; avoid being subtle. "Gosh, you have a black eye. Can you tell me how it was that you got it again?" "You said you hit your head on the corner of the desk. Tell me more about how that happened."

When physical abuse is going on, the in-laws should stay involved directly in the family and the marriage. It is amazing how much abuse continues because people have an idea that the abuse is none of their business, or they do not want to get involved.

Help from others is clearly called for.

There is a time to stand up and be counted among those who will not tolerate abuse. Do not be like one client who commented, when he heard his brother-in-law was hitting his sister, "If she did not like to be hit, she would put a stop to it." I had to explain to my client that victims of abuse, through long periods of self-denial, are often also victims of the hostage syndrome, where the person held hostage begins to identify with, and even protect, those withholding his or her personal freedom. Your help may be clearly called for, even if you risk alienating yourself from the battering in-law.

When people are abusing drugs or alcohol, they often fall down or physically injure themselves. You might want to question whether physical abuse is occurring together with substance abuse; the two often go together. Abusers and their victims need counseling and they need to make contracts with family members that they will not physically abuse. If the abuse continues, in-laws should be moved out of the home and given a safe place to stay. After people have been abused over a period of time, they may be so dispirited that they are unable to take action on their own. Under the worst of circumstances, they need to be able to go to battered women's shelters or get court-issued restraining orders.

Take it seriously when in-laws or children tell you they have been abused. Even one slap or hit is serious, and it needs to be confronted directly before it escalates into more abuse. If you have questions about your in-laws' battering, call the battered women's shelter in your area or an abuse hot line.

Even one slap or hit is serious.

Women sometimes feel that they are not abused enough to go to the battered women's shelter, but I think that if they go there for the workshops and discussion groups, it helps them to hear other people's stories about how the abuse started. If a woman is "only beaten up once a year," the threat is still there that she can be beaten up at any time, and that is a mental abuse in and of itself.

When I volunteered at the battered women's shelter in Rochester, New York, I found that 80 percent of the women who came into the shelter ultimately returned to their abusive partner. Therefore, your in-law may very well return to the person who has battered her. If you possibly can help people to work out their current battering relationships, and to set contracts for absolutely no physical abuse, it can have a positive effect because people often move from one battering relationship to another.

Everything depends on whether you can get the perpetrator to stop battering and work on the issues. If your in-law is determined to stay with the batterer ("I love him"), you might want to suggest counseling and try to get the perpetrator into a men-overcoming-violence group.

In-Law Interventions—Mildest to Most Extreme

Following are two examples of in-law problems and interventions when a family member is being abused. Alongside each are the best and worst things that might happen. Always consider possible outcomes if you intend to intervene in an in-law problem.

Make a similar chart for yourself. Be creative: Go to the extremes of the worst things that can happen. Will your in-laws never speak to you again? Will you never see your family? What will happen if you do speak up? What will happen if you do not speak up? Remember that people do not like to receive unsolicited advice from their in-laws. If you make a decision to speak up on an issue, make sure it is a critical issue. If you cry

Problem	Intervention	Best Result	Worst Result
My father-in-law harshly criticizes everything my mother-in-law does.	Get at least two family members to sit down with the father-in-law and discuss his behavior.	Father-in-law is told that the family does not support or condone his behavior and he stops doing it.	Verbal abuse continues or escalates.
My daughter-in-law beats her children with a hairbrush when they misbehave.	Parents-in-law sit down with the son- and daughter-in-law to discuss their concerns.	My daughter-in-law stops abusing the children and finds other ways to discipline them.	Children-in-law withhold having me see the grandchildren.

wolf on every issue or make cracks about everything that goes on in in-law relationships, you will lose your opportunity to be heard on the important issues and you will not have as much chance to be taken seriously.

In-Law Abuse—Overview

When has an in-law stepped over the line of what you consider acceptable behavior? What is the boundary between an occasional angry outburst and genuine abuse? It can be hard to determine, because some in-laws claim they have never had an argument with their partner or abuser, yet you have witnessed explosive temper tantrums and in-law abuse. People have differing degrees of tolerance, and it can be difficult to determine when you should step in and seek action. If you suspect that abuse might be happening, discuss it with other family members, or enlist a professional's help. If you suspect abuse and do not speak up, you are facilitating the abuser and enabling the abuse to continue. Here are some questions you might consider if you suspect that an in-law or another loved one is being abused.

Worksheet

1. Do I see any signs of physical abuse, such as bruises, black eyes, dental damage, scratches, or difficulty walking?

2. Is the abuse victim isolated from the extended family? Has this person become withdrawn?

3. Has this person stopped confiding in other family members about his or her problems or life?

4. Have there been dramatic changes in behavior that are otherwise unexplained? Is there a change in mood—less happy or more distant?

5. Does this person seem frightened of another family member or avoid being alone with him or her?

6. Does it seem that a family member must have alcohol at all gatherings? Does this family member drink excessive amounts of alcohol, or hide his or her drinking from others?

7. Is this person having problems at work or missing school for unexplained reasons?

8. Is it important that I intervene in this situation?

9. If I do not intervene, will there be negative consequences to the people I love?

10. Am I just being a "nosy neighbor"?

11. Am I thinking about intervening because there is a need, or for my own satisfaction, or to fulfill my own need to be heard and to put in my own two cents?

12. Can I live with the situation, or would I rather speak up and take the consequences?

13. What could be the positive consequences of my speaking up? What are the most negative things that could result?

PART FOUR

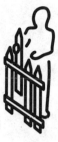

MENDING FENCES

13

Happily Ever After? Holding On to In-Law Relationships

This book is not about having perfect in-law relationships, because perfect in-law relationships are a myth. Instead, it is about how to improve and enhance your in-law relationships. As individuals, we need love and we need long-term lasting relationships. What relationships can be more significant than those we have developed with our family of origin or our in-laws?

I suggest to clients that the six letters in the word *relief* represent concept words that are keys to mending and maintaining good in-law relationships. RELIEF stands for:

R Respect

E Engagement

L Loyalty

I Initiative

E Empowerment

F Forgiveness

- **Respect:** See your in-laws as the people they are; in so doing, you will learn to respect their differences. Remember the connection that made you in-laws: You both love the same person.

- **Engagement:** Be willing to connect with your in-laws and to give them a fair hearing. In-laws bring different outlooks and opinions into the family. It is OK to agree to disagree.

- **Loyalty:** Do not expect to be called *Mom* or *Dad*. New family members sometimes feel that giving you this familial name is disloyal to their biological parents.

- **Initiative:** Take the lead in discussing and generating new options and ideas around holidays and special events. Expectations of in-laws at Thanksgiving, Christmas, Mother's Day, and Easter are hotbeds for in-law conflict. Many in-laws welcome creative alternatives.

- **Empowerment:** Honor and empower your parents-in-law by showing respect for each in-law generation. See older in-laws as experienced advisers. Honor your children-in-law by allowing them to make their own mistakes; as experienced advisers, offer unsolicited advice sparingly.

- **Forgiveness:** We all make mistakes, especially during times of change and crisis. Give up those old stories of in-law slights and rejection. It is never too late to risk a change by asking for forgiveness.

In in-law relationships, we often see patterns repeated from our own childhood.

In in-law relationships, we often see patterns repeated from our own childhood. If we can examine closely and think about our childhood relationships, we may have the key to why we have difficulty with our in-law relationships.

Resolution of in-law problems often requires employment of a variety of techniques, because of the scope of in-law problems encountered. If you have experienced an emotional or physical cutoff from your in-laws, it may take time for you to explore the cost and benefits of trying to change yourself in terms of the relationship. Take a mental inventory of how you feel about your in-laws. In the long term, the resolution of your problems may require far less energy than enduring a lifetime of continuing conflict.

Make a U-Turn to Heal In-Law Rifts

If you are at your wit's end with an in-law, think about departing from your usual solutions. What solutions have you attempted? Most of us have a range of problem-solving abilities that is not expansive. We use a few techniques over and over. Your in-laws also have a few problem-solving methods that they continually recycle.

The techniques we use are culture-bound or are learned from our own history with our in-laws. In essence, this is the monkey-see, monkey-do effect. Sometimes, when common sense and logic just do not work, why not look at the attempted solutions rather than focusing on your in-law problems? How have you tried to solve these problems? Have your solutions only added fuel to the fire?

Assess an in-law problem and make a list of what has *not* worked with this problem in the past. Then try to consider doing something different.

Consider doing something different.

When you are driving down a highway and you feel that you are not getting closer to your destination, you may realize that your direction is wrong and you need to make a complete U-turn. Is it time to take a completely different path with your in-law problem?

Dr. Richard Fisch suggests that clients identify a specific problem and then take a problem-oriented approach: List all the things that you remember your problem in-law has said. Can you come up with a common theme? Do you find that most of your problems with your in-laws arise from what is said verbally? The common theme may be: "You're not spending enough time with us" (meaning "My biological child is not spending enough time with me") or "You're not doing enough for us." Try to determine what the themes are. They usually are linked to a statement that you should be doing something, or you should stop doing something, or you should feel (or stop feeling) something. This could be called the tyranny of the shoulds—sometimes we just *should* our in-laws to death. Ask yourself what you have been doing that has contributed to this problem. Try this: After you list all the statements that start with "You should," insert "not" after each "should": "You should not do this anymore." "You should not drive me to the grocery store."

Take a chance on doing something different. Your solution may seem naive or even a bit dangerous. One of the stumbling blocks to resolution is that an in-law with whom you are having problems learns what to anticipate from you because you keep getting angry about the same kinds of things. Try to catch this in-law off guard. Try to be unpredictable—not in a mean-spirited way, but in a kind way. Rather than saying, "Why weren't you here on time yesterday?" you might say, "Gosh, you must have a really busy life. I know it is tough with little kids."

Think about the problem with that in-law. Do you think the in-law is doing it on purpose? Does it make you angry? Do you feel that the in-law is sick? Do you think the problem is superficial? Do you want a challenge, or do you feel that the in-law wants a challenge? Do you feel like a victim? Is there martyrdom? Is there devotion? Try not to think in terms of black and white. Take a look at your own attitude and feelings. Then consider making that U-turn and see what kind of response you get.

In-Law Noise

You may wish to pay attention to what I call the *noise* of in-law relationships. In order to work on or improve in-law relationships—or even to *have* in-law relationships—there has to be certain noise: a noise pro, a noise con. People have to express differences; otherwise, there really is no relationship. Or, the relationship may be weak or passive, and not worth working on. If you want to work on your in-law relationships, you have to endure the noise of relationships. Concurrently, other people in the family have to be willing to put up with, participate in, or just passively hear the noise of in-law relationships.

One of the reasons that people may relate better with in-laws in later life, particularly if they are children-in-law, is because, around the age of 28 or 30, people recognize their mortality and the fact that all humans are frail and vulnerable. Good relationships are scarce, and the world is not a better place when we lose family members. Ongoing relationships take on more value. They are worth working on. Your relationship with your in-laws may then be moving from its infancy into an awkward adolescence. You may have to deal with your in-law's or your birth relative's lack of belief that change is happening or can happen, or that you might change.

Never throw in the towel completely on a relationship. Look at the life cycle and realize that, over time, the in-law with whom you are having problems will change or you will change. Hence, even though you may let the relationship lie fallow, be willing to pick it up at another time as you change and as you feel a changed attitude coming from your in-law.

Never throw in the towel completely on a relationship.

If you care about the relationship, postpone working on it at this time, but do not ever give up on it. Using an analogy of a farmer with overworked soil, do not sell the land or give the land away. Go back and try on occasion to add soil amendments to fertilize the land. Or, plant new crops that will bring different nutrients to the soil. Prepare it to have a good yield when the time and season are ripe.

A sense of commitment and a degree of passion are necessary for building in-law relationships. Sometimes you have to just go after what you want in life. Life does not suddenly get smooth. There is never a good time or an exactly right time to try to reconcile with estranged in-laws. Sometimes you just have to *do* it.

When you are trying to deal with an in-law, check the lines of communication. Whom does communication go through? Who is the telephone dialer in the family and who listens in on a party line? Who is the gatekeeper of the in-law relationship that you are trying to enter? This person is likely the conduit to the development of healthy in-law relationships.

Signs of In-Law Meltdown

If you are on a negative track, take heart. It is never too late to renegotiate in-law relationships. The basic nutrients for growth toward positive in-law interactions are love and respect. If these are not present, the relationship is not growing; instead, it could be in danger of "in-law meltdown." Four warning signals of potential marriage meltdown have been identified by John Gottman, a psychologist at the University of Washington, who has studied more than 2,000 married couples over two decades, and Nan Silver. We can find parallel signals in in-law relationships. Ask yourself these questions:

- Am I unduly critical of my in-laws?

- Do I make comments intended to insult my in-laws, or use hostile humor?

- Am I feeling defensive or victimized by my in-laws? In response, do my in-laws deny responsibility or make excuses?

- Am I emotionally or physically withdrawing from my in-laws?

Do I want to change?

If your answer is *yes* to any of these questions, you must ask yourself another question: Do I want to change? If the answer is again *yes*, you may want to start the change process by beginning to control your advice and criticism as an important step in healing wounds.

Shortly after Sherise married Blaine, her aunt was complaining about her own mother-in-law. Sherise told her that she felt lucky to have the best mother-in-law in the world, and the aunt replied, "Then that means she never gives you any advice." After thinking about it, Sherise realized how lucky she was. In 25 years of marriage, her mother-in-law never interfered. "Her example has really taught me how to be a good mother-in-law as my own children marry," said Sherise.

Watch out for old inner *in-law scripts*, such as righteous indignation or feeling the victim. Here are some quickly accomplished strategies that

John Gottman and Nan Silver use to help diffuse couples in conflict. These strategies can also be used in your difficult in-law situations:

- Calm down. Take time out. It takes time to rewrite your inner in-law script. Practice relaxation. Take a walk.

- Speak and listen nondefensively. Be the architect of your own thoughts. Try to be a good in-law listener. Do not try to solve all the problems. Just be available.

- Validate your in-laws. Let them know that you appreciate them. Practice empathy. Try to put yourself in their shoes.

- If at first you don't succeed, try, try again.

The Good-Enough In-Law

One father-in-law said, "I really can't stand my daughter-in-law; she is ruining our grandson and I wish they would get divorced." I asked him to think about what a divorce would mean. "Number one, your daughter-in-law would still be involved with your family through your son and grandson. Number two, you and your son would have to deal with all the problems of divorce, including visitation, missing holidays, and child support, along with the loss, depression, anger, and hurt that go along with divorce." He agreed that there was enough divorce in the world, and said, "If a couple no longer wants to live together, that is one issue, but for me to put energy into seeing the marriage fail would be misplaced judgment, unless there was physical or emotional abuse." The father-in-law decided that although his daughter-in-law was not raising her son in the same way he would, she was a good wife to her husband. He said he could accept her as a "good enough in-law," even though she was not perfect.

Take a look at what a divorce would mean.

A client, Debbie, told me her sister-in-law was a control freak—she came to their apartment, and immediately began washing the dishes in the sink, *to help out*. Debbie said, "We had invited her over for eggnog, not for a scrub-down."

After acknowledging Debbie's feelings that her sister-in-law was in a territory dispute, Debbie admitted that she could put up with the "anal behavior," as she termed it, and that she actually enjoyed her sister-in-law's organizational abilities. Debbie said, "I always expect her to be perfect because she does everything so well, but that same trait can also be what turns me off when it reflects on my own housekeeping abilities. Overall, she is a great sister-in-law."

What Happens If We Do Not "Click"? When You Hate Your In-Law

"What happens if I just do not *click* with my in-laws?" Sometimes, the reason has nothing to do with you as an individual, but springs from expectations patterned into the relationship.

Your negative attitude toward an in-law may be related to a past experience with another person of the same sex, gender, or age. A young woman with whom I associate on occasion has had a difficult time with her mother. I assume her coldness toward me is related to the fact that I bear some resemblance, in age or physical characteristics, to her mother, because my encounters with this young woman have been very intermittent and her attitude toward me is unduly cool. Similar prejudices will be present when in-laws are trying to learn to relate with and integrate a new member into the family.

Pawll Lewicki, of the University of Tulsa, has shown that the unconscious mind can be biased against certain individuals when computer-generated faces are shown and it is stated that these faces are fair or unfair. In one session, Lewicki found that 20 percent of students reacted to certain individuals with bias that they were unable to explain. Their bias was learned through association with the computer-generated faces, not through actual human contact. In therapy, we call this displacement or projection: attributes or personal anger are transferred to perception of another person.

What if you really do not like your daughter- or son-in-law? What if you hate your spouse's parents? If this is the case, I suggest that you investigate whether you are dealing with one or more of the following hidden in-law agendas:

Some in-law agendas are hidden.

- In-laws who feel they know how others should behave and strive for perfection.

- In-laws who need to be the center of attention.

- In-laws who are always looking for special recognition of their achievements.

- In-laws who want you to recognize them as special, unique, and one-of-a-kind people.

- In-laws who like spending time alone and are highly protective of their time, money, and energy.

- In-laws who scan for danger in order to avoid being slighted by others.

- In-laws who concentrate on keeping the maximum number of options open.

- In-laws who have a need to be seen as in-charge individuals.

- In-laws who want to make sure family members, including in-laws, are treated fairly, thus avoiding conflict.

We all have hidden agendas; sometimes they are even hidden from ourselves. If you feel that your in-laws have a hidden agenda, see whether your own agenda conflicts. If the agendas are at odds—you both want to be in charge of the family outings—a compromise might be in order. If the agendas do not conflict, identify, acknowledge, and even learn to appreciate the in-law difference. You might find common ground by agreeing to disagree.

Relating on the Biological Plane

Did you ever stop to think about whether you're failing to click with your in-laws not only on an intellectual plane but on a biological plane as well?

Jacques, a 45-year-old librarian, told me that he loved his father-in-law but his wife's brother drove him around the bend. "He is mentally ill, does not take care of his basic hygiene, and although I know I should be sympathetic, I am tired of him ruining my carefully planned holiday gatherings," said Jacques. The brother-in-law monopolized the entire sofa because nobody could stand his odor, and then he would belch and cough all over the serving dishes at the dinner table. "I finally had to tell my father-in-law that we'd like to invite just him, and that he shouldn't just assume that we're also inviting my brother-in-law," Jacques explained. "I know it hurt his feelings that we were excluding my brother-in-law, but because of my strong feelings, I thought it better to do this so that we would not reach the point that we couldn't include my father-in-law either."

The most ancient root of our emotional life is our sense of smell.

In *Emotional Intelligence,* Daniel Goleman reminds us that the most ancient root of our emotional life is our sense of smell. Helen E. Fisher, in *Anatomy of Love,* calls this sense of smell *odorlures.* In describing why men and women become infatuated with each other, Fisher, who is a research associate in the Department of Anthropology at the Museum of Natural History, states that individuals have *apocrine* glands in their armpits, around their nipples, and in their groin, and these glands can spark strong physical and psychological reactions.

One client told me, "I like my sister-in-law but she really is hygienically challenged." The sister-in-law was an environmental activist who was concerned about not polluting the atmosphere. She chose not to use underarm deodorants, which she saw as "unnatural." Attractions and repulsions are primarily focused around love, courtship, and marriage. However, I think bending these ideas toward in-laws is useful, because different cultures express these behaviors in different ways.

Psychologist John Money, in *Love and Love Sickness: The Science of Sex, Gender Difference, and Pair-Bonding,* discusses the idea of love maps. He thinks that young children develop patterns of what feels comfortable or uncomfortable regarding physical behavior, smells, touches, jokes, and physical movements. The child then develops ideas of what is associated with disturbing experiences and what is associated with pleasant experiences. These love maps vary from one individual to another. What one person finds appealing, another person may not.

For instance, one daughter-in-law may find her father-in-law's quiet manner reassuring; another daughter-in-law may view the same manner as rejection. One son-in-law might wonder why his mother-in-law is so heavy and see her as constantly baking and pushing food on guests; another son-in-law may find this behavior nurturing.

We really need to look at our in-laws, with a biopsychosocial eye. Biologically, we are connected with our in-laws through a bond between two partners. But, human bonds, and replication of the species, are strong biological connections that bring in social issues, such as getting along with people who are not of our clan.

Strong biological connections also bring in social issues.

If you do not click with your in-laws, is it because you have had past unpleasant experiences with people of this "type"? "My father-in-law reminds me a lot of my own father, with his overdemanding way" or "My mother-in-law whines a lot, just like my mother." Here are some questions to ask yourself if you are having trouble getting along with your in-laws:

- Is the conflict really about this in-law, or am I bringing in some past family history?

- Do we smell differently or is there something about his or her body shape or the way my in-law moves that I find annoying?

- Am I sitting in judgment of my in-law, or do I think he or she is sitting in judgment of me?

- Can I find any common ground with this in-law?

- Does this in-law have any redeeming virtues?

- Do I really want to get along with this in-law, or do I just enjoy expressing some anger?

- Is my behavior with this in-law appropriate?

- Am I at least willing to agree to disagree and live and let live?

- What price do I pay for not clicking with this in-law?

- Am I dealing with a cultural issue or a personality issue?

- By not getting along with this in-law, what kind of a role model am I providing for my children?

If you care enough about your in-law to have read this entire list of questions, the situation must bother you. I would predict that after you have thoughtfully isolated some of the issues that might be causing problems, you will be 80 percent better off in your relationship with the in-law. The other 20 percent of energy can be used on some of the techniques offered throughout this book: reauthoring the stories about this in-law; identifying differences in personality types; and maintaining appropriate boundaries with a difficult in-law; or approaching this in-law in an assertive way if you feel that things may need to be handled directly.

The Dream In-Law List

Have you found yourself feeling disappointed with your in-laws because they do not live up to your expectations? Your disappointment can cause a sense of loss that may be manifested with either apathy or anger toward the in-law. If this is your status, try doing an in-law inventory of your hopes and dreams for the in-law relationship. What were your *specific* expectations? "They would have come over every Sunday for dinner," "We would have played cards," or "They would have spent family vacations with us." The first step is to write these expectations down, creating what might be called *The Dream In-Law List*.

The second step is to have family members list what they have lost because of the emotional absence or physical absence of the *ideal* in-law relationship. Ask an in-law to list how he or she would like the situation to change, or what it would take to compensate for the loss. Keep the changes simple and realistic.

What does your *real* sister-in-law, not the dream sister-in-law, have to offer at this point? What can you offer her? What might you have to give up in order to offer her the things you were ready to give to the dream sister-in-law? Would you have to give up pride, fear, anger, resentment?

List what the in-law contributes to the family.

The third step is to list what the in-law contributes to the family and what you like about him or her. This may be hard. When people are angry or hurt, they naturally defend against these feelings by being critical. Remember, the purposes of this exercise are: to deal with the loss and disappointment of a dream in-law, and to move on to more realistic expectations.

Here is how such a list might look:

Dream In-Law List	Emotional and Physical Losses to the Family of the In-Law	Contributions Made by Real In-Law	Realistic Goals
1. To play Scrabble™ together every Sunday night.	1. Realize that my brother-in-law will not stay at our house during Christmas.	1. Always helps with the cabin each spring.	1. I will make an effort to get together with my brother-in-law at least once during the holidays.
2. Take a cruise to Alaska together.	2. Realize that my sister-in-law isn't going to be my best friend.	2. Sense of humor and easy laugh help ease tense situations.	2. I will work on giving my sister-in-law some space.
3. Stay up all night and talk.			

Sooner or later, you will have to face the fact that your in-laws are not going to be the dream family that you thought you had married into. But this is not a nightmare family either; the give-and-take you can live with will be somewhere in between. Do not throw out all the good things that your in-law family has to offer you. Look within yourself: Have you been a dream in-law toward them?

Did I Tell You the One about the . . . ?

Sometimes, lack of communication with in-laws is not the problem. Too much communication can also muddy the in-law waters, especially when in-laws insist on communicating only via monologues. An in-law who binges on monologues is not responding to others' ideas or opinions. He or she seem incapable of having a two-way conversation.

To deal with an in-law who specializes in monologues, you might excuse yourself, or set a limit on how long you will listen. You could always yawn, but the monologuer probably would not notice. One of the most effective ways to deal with a person who is displaying behavior that you do not enjoy is to compliment him or her at the rare and unique times when the offensive behavior is *not* displayed. Reinforce your support of this other type of behavior by making such comments as, "Gee, thanks for listening to me. It really feels good to have you *listen*." Reinforce positive, not negative behavior.

Let's Get Rid of Those Tired Old In-Law Jokes

Comedians have harvested countless guffaws at the expense of the in-law relationship.

The in-law jokes and stories we all tell say a great deal about what our culture thinks about in-laws. Nearly all of the classic comedians have harvested countless guffaws at the expense of the in-law relationship. In *Milton Berle's Private Joke File*, the only in-law mentioned is the mother-in-law, and the majority of jokes are aimed at either getting rid of her or limiting her interference in the family's life. Here are a few examples: "I bought my mother-in-law a nice new chair—she won't plug it in." "Some airlines have a mother-in-law flight. It's non-stop."

Jokes that denigrate members of minority groups have disappeared from socially sensitive circles. Why not ditch the old mother-in-law jokes and stories too, especially when people's actual experiences with their own in-laws refute the animosity projected by in-law stories and jokes? At best, the stereotype calls forth a prejudiced response; at worst, it adversely burdens the new in-law relationship with strains and stresses arising directly from an anticipation of trouble that may be totally unwarranted.

Many of the old stereotypes about in-laws are just not true. By renouncing the old jokes and reauthoring the stories, we can make positive changes in in-law relationships. Those who would become better in-laws should refrain from telling the old jokes and from encouraging those who do. The use of labels erects barriers between in-laws. In-laws are individuals; they have their own needs, interests, and habits. The better understood, the more understandable the in-law behavior will be. When we understand people, we can learn to love and respect them.

Derogatory jokes directed toward mothers-in-law reflect the fact that, as keepers of the kin, mothers-in-law pay a heavy price. Without exception, the mother-in-law jokes are woven around a core of hostility and have familiar themes: "She talks too much," "She stays too long," "She is a meddlesome troublemaker." An analysis of marriage wit revealed that, in nearly all husband–wife jokes, women are the butt of the hostile humor. This kind of wit tends to support primarily traditional views of patriarchal control. In therapy, many couples report ongoing tensions early in their marriage that they now attribute to a preconceived idea that their mother-in-law would be a meddlesome troublemaker and should be avoided at all costs.

As keepers of the kin, mothers-in-law pay a heavy price.

The stories and jokes we use can promote or undermine individuals as well as family relationships. In-law jokes are not, however, without their benefits. Anthropologists studying kinship relationships found that joking and avoidance help in-laws to reduce potential conflict. The points of conflict that arise in relationships pose the greatest threat to loyalty, and the continued existence of mother-in-law jokes confirms an underlying tension associated with this kinship role.

Reauthoring Outmoded Stories and Stereotypes

Have you been guilty of promoting in-law bashing by telling negative stories and jokes? You might try a technique developed by Michael White and David Epston, two therapists from Australia who practice what they call *narrative therapy*.

White and Epston have found that helping families externalize their problem, by telling their story and then recreating the story (reauthoring) in a more positive way, can have healing effects. The same process can be helpful with jokes. Families can externalize their in-law tensions by telling in-law jokes, and then rewrite or retell them with other family members or individuals in mind. The final step is to analyze how and why that retelling impacts the joke. According to White and Epston, negative stories about individuals and events can trivialize and minimize—or promote and empower—individuals. How we tell our stories gives meaning to our experience.

Writing New Scripts and Legends

You have the choice: Will you replicate or correct your family scripts?

John Byng-Hall, a British therapist, discusses family behavior in terms of scripts and legends. He says that people can choose whether to replicate or correct their family scripts. For example, your father-in-law might suddenly realize that he is treating you, his son-in-law, as rudely as he was treated by his father-in-law. He can then decide to either continue his behavior or write a new script and treat you in a kinder manner. Byng-Hall says some stories are time-honored, retold again and again, and passed down through the generations. Byng-Hall terms these stories *The Legends*. Because these legends have constantly been reedited, they will tell a new in-law something about how his or her spouse's family operates and how family members are expected to behave. Our client's in-laws had strong stories of community service. The husband's grandfather was head of the local fire department and the Red Cross chapter, and owned a small store that barely supported his growing family. In contrast, the grandfather's son and grandson are successful investment advisers and bankers. By negating the story of the grandfather, they sent a message that making money was more important and community service came in second.

Another client's legend is related to the death of her father-in-law's mother after the birth of her fifth child. Her doctor had told her not to have another child because she had a bad heart. The grandfather-in-law went ahead and "got her pregnant anyway," and for this he never forgave himself. My client's parents-in-law never forgave him either, and hence were highly critical that my client had four children in very close order. Small families and wide spacing between children had become part of the family legend and her parents-in-law expected her to observe it.

You may discover that past behaviors and practices are often outdated.

The history of your family can be significant. You may discover that past behaviors and practices that are still clung to are often outdated. There is an old story about a daughter-in-law who always cut the end off a ham before she put it in the baking pan. When her mother-in-law asked why she did it this way, the girl said, "Because my mother did." When the girl asked her mother why, she was told, "I did it that way because my mother did." The girl then went to Grandma. Grandma was amused that cutting the ham had become a tradition. She had done it only because her pan was too small for the entire ham.

How do your own family stories and scripts support and perpetuate the survival of family beliefs and patterns about in-laws? Most of us retell stories related to in-laws because we have not dealt with the real issues. This was the case with the following two in-law families.

Jim, a 50-year-old police officer, said during the therapy session, "My father-in-law does not like me and has not spoken to me for five years." When questioned further, Jim replied, "He doesn't think I'm good enough for his daughter." Jim's wife, June, then said, "Come on, Jim, tell the whole story." According to Jim, "Well, June got mad and left me and went to her folks'. I went to get her and my father-in-law wouldn't let me in the house. I went to move him out of the way and pushed him a little harder than I meant to. He fell and broke his arm, and hasn't spoken to me since."

In another family, Sue, a 31-year-old homemaker, said that she was upset because her mother-in-law would not come to stay with her. Her mother-in-law apparently "didn't feel welcome at Sue's house." Sue said that she never meant to give that message. Her mother-in-law looked dubious. When questioned further, Sue said that it had all happened a year ago. "We were all playing a very competitive game and my mother-in-law supported her son (my husband) in not letting me have my turn. So I told her to get out of my house, and now she won't stay with us."

The *real endings* of these client stories remind me of radio commentator Paul Harvey, who always concludes his program by saying, "And that's the rest of the story."

Steps to Reauthor Your In-Law Stories

We all have a grab bag full of stories and jokes about ourselves and our in-laws that we can pull out at will. Assess why you remember certain in-law stories and why your family has chosen to repeat them over the years. Now try to think of yourself as a screenwriter or book author. Here are the steps you can use to reauthor negative stories:

- Pick a least hurtful story that you would like to reauthor.

- Externalize the story by discussing it with a friend or trusted family member or by writing it out and making detailed notes. If you are an artist, draw your story.

- Ask three friends who are unfamiliar with it to listen to your story without comment.

- If you are angry at a specific in-law, look for a unique outcome. When weren't you angry at that in-law?

- Approach the persons who were involved in the original story (keeping in mind the unique outcome) and discuss their perceptions in light of the fact that you are trying to reauthor the event.

- Rewrite your story or reevaluate your art. You may find that your story has changed.

As you are journaling or writing about your family of origin, your past in-law stories, or your current in-law stories, pay close attention to your body's feelings and reactions as you write. Put your story away for a few weeks. Then reread it and see how it impacts you at that time, or compare it with the other stories that you have. Consider getting together with siblings and siblings-in-law to discuss their stories. Be very careful that you do not cause people to breach loyalties or to tell family secrets that they are not privileged to reveal.

Ask the in-law family whether they have an unwritten "ten commandments for the family." What are the things they would always do and would never do? What were your own family's ten commandments? Compare them with your in-laws'.

The Healing Balm of Forgiveness

Forgiveness is an important part of the healing process. If rifts have occurred at some point in your in-law relationship, try to effect a mutual forgiveness. Someone once said that we only really become adults when we learn to forgive our parents. We could extend that maxim to the in-law relationship as well. In-laws—and people in general—seem to want forgiveness prematurely. Forgiveness is a process, not an event. You should not expect to receive instant forgiveness if you have made mistakes.

Forgiveness is a process, not an event.

The advice to "forgive and forget" is heavily laden with denial. To forgive and *remember* is a more functional strategy. Remembering will help you to identify and avoid in the future situations that breed in-law conflicts and problems. Healing is a process. Go slowly, and fully integrate changes into your life. It takes time to deal with loyalty issues, as well as feelings of hurt, exclusion, and misunderstanding.

Emotional Baggage from the Past

Few people can be always emotionally even-tempered with in-laws. When you do dump something on in-laws, or get overly angry with them because of a happening connected to your childhood, own up to the real trigger: "Look, I'm sorry I overreacted. It really wasn't about you. It was about me and some things that have gone on in my own life." Be clear about whose baggage you are carrying around.

The old saying, "Do it once, shame on you, but put up with it more than once, shame on me," means you can probably get away with blowing up at an in-law once or twice, but after that you will become *persona non grata* with that in-law. Just saying "Sorry, I have a really bad temper" is not enough. If you recognize that you have a bad temper, do something about it, or in-laws will avoid you and choose not to be in your presence.

If you plan to approach an in-law to ask for forgiveness or to solve a problem, try using my five Ds:

1. **Do it in person.** Pick your place and time carefully, and decide which in-laws or family members to invite. A personal invitation is much more effective than a letter, telephone call, card, or message relayed by a spouse.

2. **Describe the in-law problem clearly.** Use a specific incident to illustrate your point. Keep the narrative simple.

3. **Define a solution.** Have some idea of how you would like to see the in-law problem solved. Try to give your in-law two or three choices.

4. **Determine a consequence of not solving the problem.** Focus on how it would benefit both you and your in-law not to suffer this consequence.

5. **Do not force the issue.** After you have made your case, give your in-law time to consider what you have said.

One woman had, 15 years earlier, told her oldest son that his future wife was not good enough for him. In the ensuing years, somehow the wife found out, and there was still tension around this issue. My client had queried her son, and he verified that her comments made prior to their marriage were the problem. I suggested she try the five Ds of dealing with in-law problems. We then outlined the following program for her to use when she approached her daughter-in-law:

1. **Do it in person.** When I see them at Thanksgiving, I will ask my daughter-in-law if she and I can get together for lunch during the Christmas holidays. I will make a reservation for a quiet table at Green's Restaurant.

2. **Describe the in-law problem clearly.** I will say: "I would like to admit something to you. I did not know what a fine daughter-in-law you would be when Dick called to say he was going to marry you and I told him I did not think you were good enough for him. I made a mistake over 15 years ago, and I am sorry."

3. **Define a solution.** I will say: "I would like you to: forgive me; to give me another chance; and to let me know what I can do to make up for what I said."

4. **Determine a consequence of not solving the problem.** I will then add: "I'm afraid if we cannot work this out we will continue to have a tense relationship for another 15 years, which would make me very sad. I think it is also bad for the children to see their mother and grandmother not getting along."

5. **Do not force the issue.** The next time I see my daughter-in-law will be next summer. I hope we will be less tense around one another.

Mending Relationships to Create a Circle of Love and Friendship

Positive in-law relationships that have been cultivated and nurtured can create an atmosphere of love and friendship that can be very powerful, particularly in times of stress and need. The larger the circle, the more power available to stave off problems. The better your relationships with in-laws and extended family, the closer you can be and the more love and support you can receive in times of need.

A Ripple Effect

Taking responsibility for your part is a good beginning for change.

Taking responsibility for your own part in the in-law problem is a good beginning for change. If one person in the family makes a change, it creates a ripple effect of positive in-law energy and offers a role model for change. As mentioned earlier in this book, new in-laws bring in the voice of change. As a newcomer, you can often see where the in-laws are having problems. If in-laws want to change a relationship, you can give them the opportunity to see the problem in a different light. Change happens slowly. Problems build up over years, and it takes time to break down the interconnected barriers and walls. The most important underlying component for change is your *desire* to be a helping, caring, and loving in-law.

Progress, Not Perfection

When trying to change your behavior toward in-laws, give yourself permission to make a few mistakes; acknowledge that you are not perfect.

Even if the changes you are trying to make are accomplished more clumsily than you would like, if they are made with the right attitude and they help to develop closeness, love, and tolerance, you can work through the rough in-law spots.

Everyone experiences relationship problems, so it is only natural that you would experience relationship problems with your in-laws. If you do not have any relationship problems with your in-laws, you are probably not really connecting with them or you have a very superficial relationship.

Honoring the Extended Family

I believe in the old saying: "To know someone is to love them." The more you learn about the extended in-law family—its history, accomplishments, attitudes, opinions, and gender issues—the more you will come to understand why your in-laws hold the opinions that they do. It is popular today to talk about dysfunctional families, but there are really no such families. Some families, because of their problems and challenges, had to find a different way of coping than the so-called *normal* families. At one time, patterns were built up to protect the family, but these patterns may be obsolete in the 1990s. If so, in-laws, along with other interested family members, can help the family move to a higher level of coping by understanding and honoring family differences. Do not give up on the in-laws. Take the opportunity to get to know them better. You, as an in-law, can make a difference.

14

Your In-Law Inventory

Section I: In-Law History

Think back to your childhood. Many in-law problems you experience today have origins in your childhood experiences of how your parents dealt with *their* in-laws. History does not necessarily dictate your in-law destiny; however, research shows that role models—whether negative or positive—impact our behavior. What you learned about in-laws from your parents is likely to reappear in your relationship with your in-laws.

Complete this inventory in terms of you and your extended family. Read each set of instructions carefully; the point values for *Never*, *Sometimes*, and *Always* are not the same throughout. Give each issue your initial response; do not get hung up analyzing which of several in-laws it could apply to.

Alongside each of the items below, circle one number—1, 2, or 3—to indicate the appropriate response for your personal situation. Your answer should be:

       ① If this *never* happened.

       ② If this *sometimes* happened.

       ③ If this *always* happened.

	Never	Sometimes	Always

Part A

1. Did your spouse get along well with his or her parents? — 1   2   3

	Never	Sometimes	Always
1. Did your spouse get along well with his or her parents?	1	2	3
2. Do you get along well with your own parents?	1	2	3
3. Did your parents successfully resolve conflicts with their in-laws?	1	2	3
4. Were love and encouragement expressed between your parents and their in-laws?	1	2	3
5. Did your parents receive emotional, physical, or financial support from their in-laws?	1	2	3
6. Do you think that your parents truly liked their in-laws?	1	2	3
7. Did your parents' in-laws (your grandparents) support your parents with their parenting skills, including discipline?	1	2	3
8. Did your parents' in-laws express pride in your family?	1	2	3
9. Did your parents' in-laws communicate or visit often with your parents and your family?	1	2	3
10. Was your family welcome in the homes of your extended family?	1	2	3
11. Did your extended family tolerate or enjoy each other's differences?	1	2	3
12. Did your parents care enough about the extended family to be interested in and aware of the personal accomplishments and failures of their in-laws?	1	2	3
13. Was your family able to willingly support infirm or disabled in-laws?	1	2	3

	Never	Sometimes	Always
14. Did your family look forward to the holidays and vacations as a time for the extended family to be together?	1	2	3
15. Were resources of time, money, or energy shared among your extended family without expectations of exact reciprocation?	1	2	3

Add the scores you circled in each column and record the subtotals here. _____ _____ _____

Total Score Part A _____

	Never	Sometimes	Always
Part B			
1. When you were growing up, did one or both of your parents express bad feelings toward their parents-in-law?	1	2	3
2. When you were growing up, did one or both of your parents express bad feelings toward their brothers-in-law or sisters-in-law?	1	2	3
3. Was in-law bashing a favorite sport in your home during your early years?	1	2	3
4. Did your parents constantly receive advice or criticism from their in-laws?	1	2	3
5. Was your family cut off (geographically or emotionally) from in-laws?	1	2	3
6. Were there money issues with in-laws (in-laws asking for money, or loans unpaid)?	1	2	3
7. Did in-laws (your grandparents) undermine your parents' authority?	1	2	3
8. Was there competition or rivalry among the in-laws?	1	2	3

	Never	Sometimes	Always
9. Was there unresolved tension or friction between your mother and her mother-in-law (your father's mother)?	1	2	3
10. Did your parents fail to receive approval or permission to marry from their in-laws?	1	2	3
11. Was sexual, physical, or emotional abuse present in your extended family?	1	2	3
12. Were there family secrets revolving around in-laws or from which in-laws were excluded?	1	2	3
13. Did in-laws present conflicts over family holidays?	1	2	3
14. Was alcoholism or substance abuse present in your extended family?	1	2	3
15. Did your parents have clashes involving feelings of loyalty between their parents and their in-laws?	1	2	3

Add the scores you circled in each column and record the subtotals here. _____ _____ _____

Total Score Part B _____

Total Score Part A _____
less
Total Score Part B − _____
equals
Total Score Section I = _____

Section II: How Are You Treated by Your In-Laws?

Following are 50 areas of potential in-law conflict, those annoying behaviors that can drive you crazy. Recognizing that you have no control over the way others behave is the first step toward building healthy relationships with your extended family. However, it is helpful to identify those points of conflict that occur most often, in order to examine your own role in the behavior. The topics here can apply either to a specific in-law or to in-laws in general. Do not spend a lot of time analyzing the issues—your initial response will be the most telling.

Alongside each of the items below, circle one number—1, 2, or 3—to indicate the appropriate response for your personal situation. Your answer should be:

      ① If this *always* happens.

      ② If this *sometimes* happens.

      ③ If this *never* happens.

Add the numbers you circle and record the subtotals and total at the end of this section.

My in-laws (either individually or collectively) . . .

	Always	Sometimes	Never
1. Forget or botch my name.	1	2	3
2. Do not think I am good enough for the family.	1	2	3
3. Make promises to me that they seldom keep.	1	2	3
4. Nag me to help them.	1	2	3
5. Give criticism and unsolicited advice.	1	2	3
6. Always expect more from me than I am willing to give.	1	2	3
7. Only see me because they want to spend more time with their biological family.	1	2	3
8. Borrow money and do not pay it back.	1	2	3
9. Borrow items such as tools or books and never return them.	1	2	3

		Always	Sometimes	Never
10.	Get drunk at family gatherings.	1	2	3
11.	Scream and yell at each other and the extended family.	1	2	3
12.	Expect us to spend every holiday with them.	1	2	3
13.	Expect me to visit them but never visit me.	1	2	3
14.	Insist on treating and never let me reciprocate.	1	2	3
15.	Criticize how I raise my children.	1	2	3
16.	Criticize my grandparenting of their children.	1	2	3
17.	Never do anything for me.	1	2	3
18.	Say negative things about my family.	1	2	3
19.	Do not let me see my grandchildren enough.	1	2	3
20.	Only call me when they want something from me.	1	2	3
21.	Did not plan for retirement and now expect me to support them.	1	2	3
22.	Only call me when they want me to baby-sit.	1	2	3
23.	Are not willing to give me emotional support.	1	2	3
24.	Are not willing to give me physical support.	1	2	3
25.	Are not willing to give me financial support.	1	2	3
26.	Are physically abusive.	1	2	3
27.	Are sexually abusive.	1	2	3
28.	Are emotionally abusive.	1	2	3

	Always	Sometimes	Never
29. Expect to be invited on all my vacations and holidays.	1	2	3
30. Did not give permission/approval to marry their child or sibling.	1	2	3
31. Are in competition with me and each other.	1	2	3
32. Are unfair in the distribution of their resources—they give more to other in-laws than they give to me.	1	2	3
33. Think they are better than I am.	1	2	3
34. Flaunt their material possessions.	1	2	3
35. Care more about their pets than they do about me.	1	2	3
36. Care more about food than they do about me.	1	2	3
37. Would rather spend time cooking and cleaning than visiting with me.	1	2	3
38. Are consistently late to every gathering.	1	2	3
39. Change plans for every family event to fit their own agenda.	1	2	3
40. Monopolize every conversation with the same old stories and jokes.	1	2	3
41. Have unaddressed gender issues that get taken out on me.	1	2	3
42. Are unwilling to consider another viewpoint.	1	2	3
43. Whine or complain about minor details.	1	2	3
44. Spend too much money on me and then act like they own me.	1	2	3
45. Expect my spouse to be their handyman or housemaid and then do			

	Always	Sometimes	Never
not show appreciation or offer him or her compensation.	1	2	3
46. Belittle my spouse.	1	2	3
47. Think I drink too much.	1	2	3
48. Do not like my life priorities.	1	2	3
49. Think they know what is right or wrong and expect everyone to agree.	1	2	3
50. Are indecisive and expect me to make all the decisions.	1	2	3
Subtotals	_____	_____	_____
Total Score Section II	_____		

Section III: How Do You Feel about Your In-Laws?

You cannot change others, but you can change yourself. This part of the inventory explores your feelings, attitudes, and reactions toward in-laws. Your answers will indicate how you are as an in-law and will identify the potential problem areas where you may wish to focus your attention. The topics can apply either to a specific in-law or to in-laws in general. Do not spend a lot of time analyzing the issues—your initial response will be the most telling.

Alongside each of the items below, circle one number—1, 2, or 3—to indicate the appropriate response for your personal situation. Your answer should be:

① If this *never* happens.

② If this *sometimes* happens.

③ If this *always* happens.

Add the numbers you circle and record the subtotals and total at the end of this section.

	Never	Sometimes	Always
Around my in-laws (either individually or collectively), I . . .			
1. Am comfortable and feel like I can be myself.	1	2	3
2. Feel support.	1	2	3
3. Receive positive feedback.	1	2	3
4. Feel that my opinion is respected.	1	2	3
5. Feel welcomed and considered a member of the clan.	1	2	3
6. Received permission/approval to marry my spouse.	1	2	3
7. Am trusted.	1	2	3
8. Feel free to ask for help.	1	2	3
9. Feel like they appreciate my interests and accomplishments.	1	2	3
10. Am not punished for taking time-out and have the freedom to pursue my own interests.	1	2	3
11. Am appreciated for my contributions.	1	2	3
12. Feel appreciated for my unique personality and the difference I bring to the family.	1	2	3
13. Am listened to.	1	2	3
14. Am invited to family gatherings.	1	2	3
15. Am given the option to decline invitations without risk of hurt feelings.	1	2	3
16. Feel like I am friend with my in-laws.	1	2	3
17. Enjoy spending holidays together.	1	2	3
18. Feel healthy and happy.	1	2	3
19. Find my extended family relationship satisfying.	1	2	3

		Never	Sometimes	Always
20.	Know they would help in a financial pinch.	1	2	3
21.	Could depend on them if I were ill.	1	2	3
22.	Can request assistance with transportation.	1	2	3
23.	Can ask for baby-sitting.	1	2	3
24.	Can decline to baby-sit without hurting their feelings.	1	2	3
25.	Can have a beer without being accused of being an alcoholic.	1	2	3
26.	Can receive criticism from them without taking offense.	1	2	3
27.	Feel good about helping when they are in trouble.	1	2	3
28.	Enjoy organizing family events.	1	2	3
29.	Enjoy pitching in when the extended family gets together.	1	2	3
30.	Look forward to family events.	1	2	3
31.	Would like it if they lived closer to me.	1	2	3
32.	Enjoy taking short trips or vacations.	1	2	3
33.	Like to go to the movies or out to lunch.	1	2	3
34.	Enjoy golfing or other outdoor activities.	1	2	3
35.	Like to use my talents to help them.	1	2	3
36.	Enjoy selecting or making gifts for them.	1	2	3
37.	Enjoy just sitting down and talking with them.	1	2	3
38.	Find them interesting and enjoy hearing their opinions.	1	2	3
39.	Do not mind it when they repeat themselves.	1	2	3

		Never	Sometimes	Always
40.	Think they are amusing and say the funniest things.	1	2	3
41.	Appreciate the new circle of friends they have introduced me to.	1	2	3
42.	Enjoy looking at photo albums, slides, or home videos and hearing about their family history.	1	2	3
43.	Think it is nice knowing someone else cares about my spouse and kids as much as I do.	1	2	3
44.	Feel thankful that they can pinch-hit for me when I am out of town.	1	2	3
45.	Am glad that in an impersonal world there are still strong personal relationships.	1	2	3
46.	Know that they will support me in my child-rearing efforts.	1	2	3
47.	Am encouraged to be the best I can be.	1	2	3
48.	Receive financial assistance with no strings attached.	1	2	3
49.	Can be wrong and be forgiven.	1	2	3
50.	Can forgive and forget the hurts and insults I receive.	1	2	3

Subtotals ____ ____ ____

Total Score Section III ____

Section IV: Your Willingness to Change

How willing are you to make changes in the way you deal with your in-laws? The most important underlying component for change is your *desire* to be a helping, caring, and loving in-law. Coupled with this desire, you need flexibility and a willingness to change. Relationships are fluid, and a willingness to make some of the simple changes outlined below can free up energy and creativity for the entire family. The following questions will indicate your willingness to change. Do not spend a lot of time analyzing the issues—your initial response will be the most telling.

Alongside each of the items below, circle one number—1, 2, or 3—to indicate the appropriate response for your personal situation. Your answer should be:

① *No* (I am unwilling to change).

② *Maybe* (I will consider changing).

③ *Yes* (I will definitely change).

Add the numbers you circle, and record the subtotals and total at the end of this section.

Will I . . .	No	Maybe	Yes
1. Try to remain neutral in family disputes?	1	2	3
2. Give advice sparingly and only when asked?	1	2	3
3. Be a flexible in-law and accept differences?	1	2	3
4. Offer my in-laws a helping hand?	1	2	3
5. Maintain a sense of humor?	1	2	3
6. Give my in-laws the benefit of the doubt?	1	2	3
7. Try to make it convenient for in-laws to visit the family?	1	2	3
8. Visit and be visited by in-laws without keeping count of whose turn it is?	1	2	3
9. Forgive my in-laws for past slights?	1	2	3

	No	Maybe	Yes
10. Show my children a positive in-law role model by treating my in-laws as well as I treat my friends?	1	2	3
11. Ask my spouse to deal directly with his or her family members when there is a dispute, and not involve me as an in-law?	1	2	3
12. Be satisfied to grow through small in-law successes?	1	2	3
13. Risk being converted to my in-laws' ideas?	1	2	3
14. Give my in-laws an out?	1	2	3
15. Allow some room for movement, and avoid backing them into a corner?	1	2	3
16. Learn to expect to not be appreciated?	1	2	3
17. Focus on what my in-laws know, rather than what they do not know?	1	2	3
18. Be willing to reinvent the wheel and change in-law relationships?	1	2	3
19. Model what I want—behave in the way I would like to be treated?	1	2	3
20. Respect the in-laws' past, acknowledging that before I came into the family, there were relationships and there was a family organization?	1	2	3
Subtotals	____	____	____
Total Score Section IV			____

Section V: What Your In-Law Inventory Means

The best gift you can give yourself and your extended family is a happy in-law, and the only in-law whom you can guarantee will be happy is you.

Take the time to analyze yourself as an in-law and to explore your needs, your in-law desires, and what is going on between you and your in-laws.

At some point in your life, you have to ask yourself, "How far am I willing to reach out to the extended family?" Only you can answer this question, and you hold within yourself the ability to bring about positive change in your entire family. As you work through your in-law problems, remember the ripple effect—change that is effected by just one person will, by its very nature, create change throughout the entire family.

Now, add the totals from each of the sections:

	Totals
Section I: In-Law History	_____
Section II: How Are You Treated by Your In-Laws?	_____
Section III: How Do You Feel about Your In-Laws?	_____
Section IV: Your Willingness to Change	_____
Grand Total In-Law Inventory Score	_____

Self-Evaluation

The *grand total in-law inventory score* will help you identify where you are on the spectrum of in-law relationships, and your answers to individual questions will indicate areas where change is needed. After you know your grand total, ask your spouse and your in-laws to complete the inventory. In comparing answers, you may note that totals for women will run higher than those for men. As *keepers of the kin*, women tend to be more deeply involved in relationships with the extended family.

Range of Scores

331–390   You have almost ideal in-law relationships. If others follow your example, they cannot go wrong. In fact, perhaps you should send me your tips for having an ideal in-law relationship. You and your extended family deserve to be congratulated—keep up the good work!

271–330   Even though you and your in-laws have your ups and downs, overall, you have been able to forge a healthy give-and-take with your extended family. However, note the areas that received negative scores, because these indicate potential areas of conflict and stress. Consider your role and how *you* might change, to turn the situation around in those areas.

201–270   You have had less than amicable relationships with your in-laws. But there is still hope. Try to concentrate on the inventory areas that received positive scores, and think about what you can do to repeat the success stories. Especially important for you will be the answers in Section IV. You might want to identify the areas where you circled 2s—"*Maybe* (I will consider changing)"—and do what you can to turn those answers to 3s—"*Yes* (I will definitely change)." But start slowly and build on gradual successes.

200 or fewer   You are experiencing an epic in-law disaster, and my heart goes out to you and your in-laws. Your score is a strong indicator that you need to learn new ways to deal with your in-laws and extended family. Beware of reinforcing old negative patterns. For the areas that received negative scores, beware of similar problems that can be passed down through the generations. Remember, those who do not learn from history are destined to repeat it. You may have inherited your family's genetic material, but that does not mean you are forced to carry on their unhealthy behavior patterns in your in-law relationships. If you find it hard to change on your own, consider individual therapy or family counseling.

Notes

Preface

v   Murray Bowen (1978). *Family therapy in clinical practice*. New York: Jason Aronson.

Chapter 1   What Type of In-Law Are You?

5   "In the United States today": Robert Famighetti (Ed.) (1994). *The World Almanac and Books of Facts*. Mahwah, NJ: Funk & Wagnalls.

5   Ann Cryster (1990). *The wife-in-law trap*. New York: Pocket Books.

5   Monica McGoldrick (1982). Ethnicity and family therapy: An overview. In M. McGoldrick, J. K. Pearce, and J. Giordano (Eds.), *Ethnicity and family therapy*. New York: Guilford Press.

6   Evelyn R. Duvall (1954). *In-laws, pro and con: An original study of interpersonal relations*. New York: Association Press.

6   "One of the most useful models": Helen Palmer (1988). *The Enneagram: Understanding yourself and the others in your life*. San Francisco: Harper & Row.

Chapter 2   Bad In-Laws and Good In-Laws

30   Linda Berg-Cross and Jacqueline Jackson (1986). Helping the extended family: In-law growth and development training program. *Psychotherapy in Private Practice, 4*(1), 33–50.

37   Kevin Leman (1985). *The birth order book: Why you are the way you are*. New York: Dell.

Chapter 3   Forming, Storming, Norming, and Conforming

43   Virginia Satir (1988). *The new peoplemaking*. Mountain View, CA: Science and Behavior Books.

44   Gregory Bateson (1980). *Mind and nature: A necessary unity* (p. 74). New York: Bantam.

45   "Most in-law relationships": Bruce W. Tuckman (1965). Developmental sequence in small groups. *Psychological Bulletin, 63,* 384–389; Bruce W. Tuckman and Mary Ann C. Jensen (1977). Stages of small group development revisited, *Group and Organizational Studies, 2*(4), 419–427.

49   Evelyn R. Duvall (1954).

50   Monica McGoldrick (1980). The joining of families through marriage: The new couple. In E. A. Carter and M. McGoldrick (Eds.), *The family life cycle: A framework for family therapy* (pp. 93–119). New York: Gardner.

51   Paulinia McCullough (1980). Launching children and moving on. In E. A. Carter and M. McGoldrick (Eds.), *The family life cycle: A framework for family therapy* (pp. 171–195). New York: Gardner.

Chapter 4   Marrying the Family

62   "Although some experts feel": Ivan Boszormenyi-Nagy and Geraldine M. Spark (1973). *Invisible loyalties.* New York: Brunner/Mazel.

62   Arthur L. Leader (1975). The place of in-laws in marital relationships. *Social Casework, 21,* 486–491.

64   M. Duncan Stanton (1981). Marital therapy from a structural/strategic viewpoint. In G. P. Sholevar (Ed.), *Marriage is a family affair: A textbook of marriage and marital therapy.* New York: SP Medical and Scientific Books.

Chapter 5   When Babies Enter the In-Law Picture

84   "Of this number": Lillian E. Troll, S. J. Miller, and R. C. Atchley (1979). *Being a grandparent or greatgrandparent: Families in later life.* Belmont, CA: Wadsworth.

85   "The birth of a grandchild": Nora Reiner Gluck, Elaine Dannefer, and Kathryn Milea (1980). Women in families. In E. A. Carter and M. McGoldrick (Eds.), *The family life cycle: A framework for family therapy* (pp. 295–327). New York: Gardner.

85   "But when three generations": Edith Mendel Stern (1965). *You and your aging parents.* New York: Harper & Row.

89 Helen Q. Kivnick (1982). *The meaning of grandparenthood.* Ann Arbor, MI: UMI Research Press.

90 Andrew Cherlin and Frank Furstenberg (1985). Styles and strategies of grandparenting. In V. L. Bengston and J. F. Robertson (Eds.), *Grandparenthood* (pp. 97–116). Beverly Hills, CA: Sage.

90 Lillian E. Troll (1983). Grandparents: The family watchdogs. In T. Brubaker (Ed.), *Family relationships in later life* (pp. 63–74). Beverly Hills, CA: Sage.

91 "Humorist Sam Levinson": L. M. Boyd (1995, February 23). For your information. *The Houston Post,* p. A16.

93 Evelyn R. Duvall (1954).

Chapter 6   Changing Tides—Aging and the In-Law Relationship

103 Elizabeth A. Carter and Monica McGoldrick (Eds.) (1980). *The family life cycle: A framework for family therapy.* New York: Gardner.

108 Nancy L. Mace and Peter V. Rubins (1991). *The 36-Hour day: A family guide to caring for persons with Alzheimer's disease related dementing illnesses, and memory loss in later life.* Baltimore: Johns Hopkins University Press.

108 Lenore S. Powell with Katie Courtice (1993). *Alzheimer's disease: A guide for families.* New York: Addison-Wesley.

108 *Consumer Reports,* Joel Gurin (Ed.). August, September, and October 1995. Yonkers, NY: Consumers Union.

110 "Not all adjustments": Colin Murry Parkes and Robert S. Weiss (1983). *Recovery from bereavement.* New York: Basic Books.

111 "Another important finding": Ibid.

112 James L. Framo (1992). *Family of origin therapy: An intergenerational approach.* New York: Brunner/Mazel.

112 Trudy Anderson (1984). Widowhood as a life transition: Its impact on kinship ties. *Journal of Marriage and the Family,* 46(1), 105–114.

Chapter 7   Between a Rock and a Hard Place—Dealing with Divided Loyalties

117 "In order to love yourself": Ivan Boszormenyi-Nagy and Geraldine M. Spark (1973).

118 Ibid.

120 Abraham Lincoln (1858). Springfield Speech, June 16, 1858.

122 Barbara Goulter and Joan Minninger (1993). *The father-daughter dance. Insight, inspiration, and understanding for every woman and her father.* New York: G. P. Putnam's Sons.

122 Mirra Komarovsky (1962). *Blue-collar marriage.* New York: Random House.

125 Emily Martinsen and Joyce Bolender (1995). *The troublesome triangle.* Ocala, FL: Special Publications.

126 "Fathers can often wield": Barbara Goulter and Joan Minninger (1993).

127 "Family secrets become": Fritz B. Simon, Helm Stierlin, and Lyman C. Wynne (1985). *The language of family therapy: A systematic vocabulary and sourcebook* (p. 136). New York: Family Process Press.

127 James L. Framo (1965). Rationale and techniques of intensive family therapy. In Ivan Boszormenyi-Nagy and James L. Framo (Eds.), *Intensive family therapy: Theoretical and practical aspects* (pp. 143–212). New York: Harper & Row.

129 Evan Imber-Black (1993). *Secrets in families and family therapy* (p. 4). New York: Norton.

130 John Bradshaw (1995). *Family secrets: What you don't know can hurt you.* New York: Bantam.

Chapter 8   Who's the Boss? The Struggle for Power

136 "At a recent international conference": Seminar: *In laws: Therapeutic issues and techniques for working with the extended family,* Seventh Annual World Family Therapy Conference, Guadalajara, Mexico, October 1995.

143 Evelyn R. Duvall (1954).

145 Monica McGoldrick (1980).

149 Evelyn R. Duvall (1954).

150 Paula J. Caplan (1989). *Don't Blame Mother: Mending the Mother–Daughter Relationship.* New York: Harper & Row.

151 "The most common complaints": Evelyn R. Duvall (1954).

Chapter 9   Can We Talk? Coping with Communication Problems

155 Gerald R. Weeks and Stephen Treat (1992). *Couples in treatment. Techniques and approaches for effective practice.* New York: Brunner/Mazel.

157 Michael P. Nichols (1995). *The lost art of listening*. New York: Guilford Press.

159 George R. Bosh and Peter Wyden (1968). *The intimate enemy: How to fight fair in love and marriage*. New York: Avon.

164 Linda Berg-Cross and Jacqueline Jackson (1986).

166 Linda Adams and Elinor Lenz (1989). *Be your best*. New York: Perigree. See also Manual J. Smith (1975). *When I Say No, I Feel Guilty*. New York: Bantam.

Chapter 10   The Holidays—An In-Law Adventure That Keeps on Going . . . and Going . . . and Going

169 Evan Imber-Black and Janine Roberts (1992). *Rituals for our times*. New York: HarperPerennial.

172 Linda Berg-Cross and Jacqueline Jackson (1986).

180 Wayne Dyer (1986). *No more holiday blues*. New York: Harper-Paperbacks.

185 Jo Robinson and Jean Coppock Staheli (1991). *Unplug the Christmas machine*. New York: William Morrow.

187 "Like the Japanese": Christopher Engholm (1991). *When business east meets business west: The guide to practice and protocol in the Pacific Rim*. New York: John Wiley & Sons, Inc.

Chapter 11   Money, Love, and Other Scarce In-Law Resources

194 Virginia Satir (1964). *Conjoint family therapy: A guide to theory and technique*. Palo Alto, CA: Science and Behavior Books.

201 Florence W. Kaslow (1991). Enter the prenuptial: A prelude to marriage or remarriage. *Behavioral Sciences and the Law*, 9, 375–386.

202 Ibid.

206 "Without undue delay": Robert J. Lynn (1992). *Introduction to estate planning in a nutshell* (4th ed.). St. Paul, MN: West.

208 Ibid.

208 Harry D. Krause (1986). *Family law in a nutshell* (2nd ed.). St. Paul, MN: West. See also Robert J. Lynn (1992).

209 Emily B. Visher and John S. Visher (1982). *How to win as a stepfamily* (2nd ed.). New York: Brunner/Mazel.

Chapter 12   When In-Laws Hurt the One You Love

225   "In-law loyalties": Ammy van Heusden and ElseMarie van den Eerenbeemt (1986). *Balance in motion: Ivan Boszormenyi-Nagy and his vision of individual and family therapy.* New York: Brunner/Mazel. See also Ivan Boszormenyi-Nagy and Geraldine Spark (1973).

Chapter 13   Happily Ever After? Holding On to In-Law Relationships

235   "When you are driving": Richard Fisch and Karin Schlanger (1995). Brief Therapy Intensive Training, Mental Research Institute, Palo Alto, CA.

238   John Gottman and Nan Silver (1994). *Why marriages succeed or fail.* New York: Simon & Schuster.

240   Pawll Lewicki (1992, June 23). Your unconscious mind may be smarter than you. *New York Times*, p. B5.

242   Daniel Goleman (1995). *Emotional intelligence.* New York: Bantam.

242   Helen E. Fisher (1992). *Anatomy of love: The natural history of monogamy, adultery, and divorce.* New York: Norton.

243   John Money (1980). *Love and love sickness: The science of sex, gender difference, and pair-bonding.* Baltimore: Johns Hopkins University Press.

246   Milton Berle (1989). *Milton Berle's private joke file.* New York: Crown.

247   "An analysis of marriage wit": Evelyn R. Duvall (1954).

247   "Anthropologists": Alfred R. Radcliffe-Brown (1952). *Structure and function in primitive society: Essays and addresses.* Glencoe, IL: Free Press.

248   "The points of conflict": J. Schlien (1962). Mother-in-law—A problem in terminology. *Etc.*, *19*, 161–171.

248   Michael White and David Epston (1989). *Literate means to therapeutic ends.* Adelaide, South Australia: Dulwich Centre Publications.

248   John Byng-Hall (1988). Scripts and legends in families and family therapy. *Family Process*, *27*, 167–179.